Mayo Clinic on Digestive Health

John King, M.D.

Editor in Chief

Mayo Clinic

Rochester, Minnesota

Published by Mayo Clinic Health Solutions, Rochester, Minn. For bulk sales to employers, member groups and health-related companies, contact Mayo Clinic Health Solutions, 200 First St. SW, Rochester, MN, 55905, or send an e-mail to SpecialSalesMayoBooks @Mayo.edu.

Photo credits: Cover photos from PhotoDisc

Library of Congress Catalog Card Number: 2003114860

Printed in Canada

Second Edition

4 5 6 7 8 9 10

About digestive disease

Digestive problems are among the most common reasons people see their doctors. They're also a leading reason people take medication. Each month, more than 40 percent of adults in the United States take antacids or other acid-suppressing medications to treat heartburn alone. Other common digestive complaints include indigestion, abdominal pain, nausea, diarrhea, constipation and gas. You may have come to accept these signs and symptoms as byproducts of digestion. Often, though, they're your body's way of telling you that something is wrong. The good news is that with early diagnosis, most digestive problems often can be successfully treated.

Within these pages you'll find practical advice you can use to identify and treat digestive problems, before they become difficult to manage or a threat to your life. You'll also learn about lifestyle changes that may reduce your risk of digestive disease. This book is based on the expertise of Mayo Clinic doctors and the advice they give day in and day out in caring for their patients.

About Mayo Clinic

Mayo Clinic evolved from the frontier practice of Dr. William Worrall Mayo, and the partnership of his two sons, William J. and Charles H. Mayo, in the early 1900s. Pressed by the demands of their busy practice in Rochester, Minn., the Mayo brothers invited other physicians to join them, pioneering the private group practice of medicine. Today, with more than 2,000 physicians and scientists at its three major locations in Rochester, Minn., Jacksonville, Fla., and Scottsdale, Ariz., Mayo Clinic is dedicated to providing comprehensive diagnoses, accurate answers and effective treatments.

With its depth of medical knowledge, experience and expertise, Mayo Clinic occupies an unparalleled position as a health information resource. Since 1983, Mayo Clinic has published reliable health information for millions of consumers through award-winning newsletters, books and online services. Revenue from the publishing activities supports Mayo Clinic programs, including medical education and research.

Editorial staff

Editor in Chief
John King, M.D.

Managing Editor
Richard Dietman

Editorial Research
Anthony Cook
Danielle Gerberi
Deirdre Herman
Michelle Hewlett
Stephen Johnson

Contributing Writers
Lee Engfer
Rebecca Gonzalez-Campoy
Lynn Madsen
Stephen Miller

Proofreading
Miranda Attlesey
Mary Duerson
Donna Hanson

Creative Director
Daniel Brevick

Design
Craig King

Illustration
Brian Fyffe
Steven Graepel
John Hagen
Michael King

Indexing
Larry Harrison

Contributing editors and reviewers

David Ahlquist, M.D.
David Brandhagen, M.D.
Suresh Chari, M.D.
Claude Deschamps, M.D.
Jeff Fidler, M.D.
Christopher Frye
Christopher Gostout, M.D.
Axel Grothey, M.D.
Gavin Harewood, M.D.

C. Daniel Johnson, M.D.
Giles Locke III, M.D.
Joseph Murray, M.D.
Jennifer K. Nelson, R.D.
Yvonne Romero, M.D.
Jacalyn See, R.D.
William Tremaine, M.D.
Tonia Young-Fadok, M.D.

Preface

Welcome to the second edition of *Mayo Clinic on Digestive Health*. You may have picked up this book because you're bothered by a problem such as heartburn, abdominal pain or diarrhea, and you're not sure what's causing it. Or perhaps you know what your problem is, and you're looking for how best to treat it. Maybe you're searching for a way to prevent a digestive condition. This second edition has been extensively updated with information about digestive diseases and the most recent diagnostic and treatment options. For example, there's new information on celiac disease and on a relatively new diagnostic tool called endoscopic ultrasound. There's also the latest on minimally invasive treatments for GERD and information on the new DNA stool test for colorectal cancer.

Your digestive tract is a complex system that delivers the energy and nutrients you need to live. When you consider that your digestive tract extends from your mouth to your anus and involves several essential organs, it's easy to imagine the problems that might occur there.

Nearly everyone experiences problems such as heartburn, diarrhea, constipation or abdominal discomfort at some point. But because over-the-counter medications may temporarily relieve them, many people don't see their doctors — or they wait too long. If you have recurring or persistent symptoms, don't ignore them. Early treatment can prevent a problem from becoming serious, and it increases the chance that your condition can be treated or cured.

In this book, you'll find practical, easy-to-understand information on how your digestive system works, factors that can interfere with digestion, and how to prevent digestive problems. Signs and symptoms of common digestive problems are discussed, and diagnostic procedures used to help identify the causes of digestive problems are reviewed. The rest of the book is devoted to treatment of common digestive diseases and conditions. Along with the advice of your doctor, this book can help you enjoy life with fewer digestive problems.

John King, M.D.
Editor in Chief

Contents

Chapter 1

Americans and digestion

Heartburn, cramps, nausea, diarrhea, constipation. These are just a few of the ways your stomach and intestines let you know when they aren't well. At one time or another, most people experience these signs and symptoms. Often, they last just a day or two and then disappear. But for many people, the signs and symptoms linger and become a daily challenge.

It's estimated that about one in three Americans experiences some kind of digestive difficulty and that more than 10 million are hospitalized each year for digestive problems. You can see the evidence of how common these problems are in your local drug, grocery or discount store. Shelves are lined with medicines to treat digestive conditions. These include antacids, acid blockers, laxatives, fiber supplements and antidiarrheals. Each year Americans spend more than $3 billion on these over-the-counter products.

Although they can help relieve symptoms, over-the-counter medications may not be the complete answer. If you're bothered by a digestive problem, it's important that you see your doctor. Digestive problems can occur for many reasons. By knowing the cause of your problem, you and your doctor can work together on a plan to treat your condition and possibly even cure it. Early action on your part also can prevent a serious condition from becoming life-threatening.

Lifestyle issues

Are digestive problems more common today than years ago? There aren't any figures that provide a definitive answer. However, several factors, including the popularity of over-the-counter medications, suggest this may be true.

Why are more people experiencing stomach and intestinal problems? There may be many reasons, but a likely cause is lifestyle.

Eating in a hurry. Hectic schedules have more people rushing through their meals or eating on the go. When you eat fast, you tend not to chew your food long enough or to grind it into small enough pieces. This forces your digestive system to work harder. When you gulp down food, you also swallow more air than when you eat slowly, and this leads to belching and intestinal gas.

A high-fat diet. Fast-food restaurants and prepackaged meals are popular conveniences. But fat and excess calories are often part of this type of diet. The average American eats too much fat and not enough fiber found in fruits, vegetables and grains. Fiber helps food pass smoothly through your digestive tract. Fat does the opposite. It slows digestion.

Studies also suggest that a diet high in saturated fats (animal fats) may increase your risk of cancer, especially colon cancer. Exactly how fat may contribute to cancer is unclear, but research suggests that it may promote the formation of cancer-causing substances (carcinogens).

Inactivity. Many people in the United States are becoming increasingly sedentary. Regular physical activity is important for digestion because it helps speed the movement of waste through your digestive tract in addition to helping you maintain a healthy weight.

Obesity. Too much dietary fat and too little physical activity have resulted in a dramatic increase in the the number of obese Americans. About 30 percent of American adults have a body mass index (BMI) equal to or greater than 30 and are considered obese. That means they're at least 30 percent above their healthy weight. That figure represents more than a 50 percent jump in the rate of obesity from 1960, when about 13 percent of the adult population was obese.

Excess weight is associated with a number of digestive problems. The most common is gastroesophageal reflux disease (GERD). Extra pounds increase pressure within your abdomen and in turn push on your stomach. Increased pressure on your stomach forces stomach acid back into your esophagus, causing a burning sensation in your esophagus (heartburn) and inflammation of tissues that line the esophagus (esophagitis). Excess weight also increases your risk of gallbladder disease and possibly colon cancer.

Stress. Many Americans live stressful, time-pressured lives. Your body doesn't digest food well when you're stressed. It concentrates on dealing with the stress, leaving less blood volume for other functions, such as digestion.

Smoking. Smokers are more likely to have indigestion, stomach ulcers and cancer of the esophagus. The good news is that once you stop smoking, some of these digestive problems may disappear.

Problems by the numbers

The prevalence of digestive problems is reflected in these general statistics.

- Approximately 40 percent of Americans experience heartburn at least once a month. Ten percent have heartburn weekly.
- About 50 million Americans have trouble digesting dairy products, a condition called lactose intolerance.
- An estimated 30 to 45 million Americans experience abdominal pain, gas, and diarrhea or constipation, associated with irritable bowel syndrome.
- About three million Americans say they have frequent constipation.
- About one in 10 Americans develops an ulcer at some point in his or her life.
- More than 2.7 million Americans are chronically infected with the hepatitis C virus.
- Cancer of the colon and rectum is second only to lung cancer as the leading cause of cancer-related deaths in the U.S. It takes more than 57,000 lives each year.

Alcohol. Too much alcohol can inflame your stomach lining and relax the muscular valve (lower esophageal sphincter) that seals and protects your esophagus from stomach acid. Women may be more susceptible to alcohol-related disorders because their bodies produce fewer enzymes to break down alcohol.

How digestion works

A general explanation of how digestion works may help you to understand why digestive problems are so common. Your digestive system is much more than just your stomach and intestines. It's a complex system of organs that conveys and converts the food you eat into the energy you need. Because of this, digestion is one of the most important functions your body performs.

The salivary glands

Digestion starts even before you take your first bite. The aroma of the food you're about to eat — or even the thought of eating — is enough to get saliva in your mouth flowing. In addition to smaller glands in the lining of your mouth, you have three pairs of large salivary glands, each designed for different purposes. Together, they produce about 3 pints of saliva daily.

Parotid glands. These glands are in your cheeks, just under your earlobes. Pressure from your molars, or salty or bitter food, causes these glands to excrete your most potent saliva, which contains the enzyme amylase (AM-uh-lase). This enzyme begins to convert starches into sugar. As you chew, you may actually taste the food getting sweeter. Saliva from the parotid glands also contains anti-bodies that fight bacteria.

Submandibular glands. These glands lie in the back of your mouth, along each side of your lower jawbone and deep beneath your tongue. They're activated by sour or fatty foods. They produce a thick saliva to help you swallow bulky food.

Sublingual glands. The smallest of the three pairs, these glands are located in tissue at the floor of your mouth, just below your tongue. They produce a thinner saliva, ideal for diluting sugar.

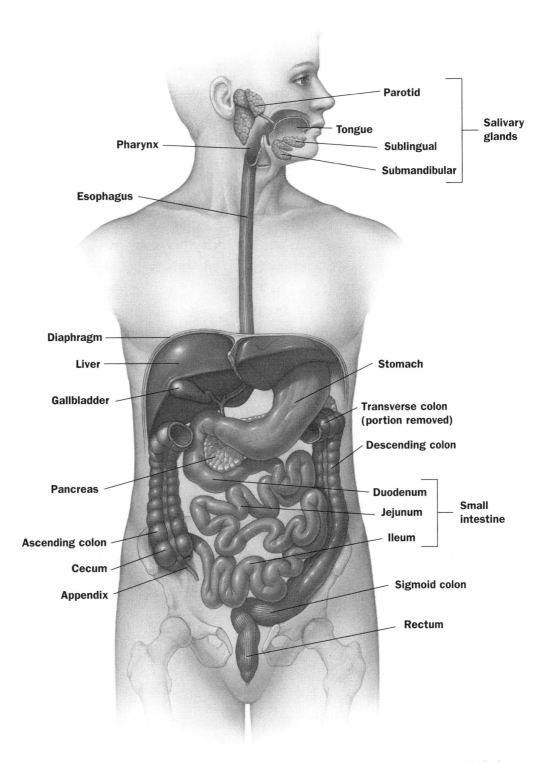

Parotid

Tongue

Sublingual

Submandibular

Salivary glands

Pharynx

Esophagus

Diaphragm

Liver

Gallbladder

Stomach

Transverse colon (portion removed)

Descending colon

Pancreas

Duodenum

Jejunum

Small intestine

Ileum

Ascending colon

Cecum

Appendix

Sigmoid colon

Rectum

The digestive tract begins at the mouth and ends at the rectum. It includes several vital internal organs.

Sublingual glands are triggered by sweet food and natural sugars in fruits and vegetables.

When you take a bite, your salivary glands kick into high gear, pumping out saliva that begins to chemically break down the food. Not all the work is chemical, though. Your teeth crunch and grind the food, while your tongue mixes it with saliva. This chewing and churning transform a bite of food into what's called a bolus — a soft, moist, rounded mixture suitable for swallowing.

The esophagus

What you put into your mouth, how long you chew it, and when you swallow, are all things you control. But once you swallow, the rest of the digestive process is controlled by your nervous system.

When you swallow, muscles in your mouth and throat propel food through a relaxed ring of muscle (upper esophageal sphincter) that connects the back of your throat (pharynx) to your upper esophagus. From there, the food passes through your esophagus, a tube typically about 10 inches long, that connects your throat and stomach. Inside your esophagus, muscles move in synchronized waves — one after another — propelling the food toward your stomach. Muscles behind the swallowed food contract, squeezing it forward, while muscles in front relax to allow the food to advance without resistance. This pattern of progressive contraction and relaxation is called peristalsis (per-ih-STAL-sis) — a process that continues through your entire digestive tract.

The muscles that line your esophagus are so strong that they can overcome gravity and send food to your stomach even if you stand on your head. This is why astronauts in zero gravity are able to eat. However, to let gravity assist in swallowing and to help prevent partially digested food from passing from your stomach up into your esophagus (gastroesophageal reflux), it's best to wait at least two to three hours after eating before lying down.

Once food reaches the lower portion of your esophagus, it approaches the lower esophageal sphincter. When you're not eating, this muscle valve remains tightly closed to keep stomach acid from flowing backward (regurgitating) into your esophagus and causing heartburn. Pressure from food in the esophagus signals this muscle valve to relax and open to let the food pass through on its way to your stomach.

The stomach

Your stomach sits in the upper left corner of your abdomen, just under your rib cage. A hollow, muscular sac, the typical stomach is about 10 inches long and can expand at the sides to hold about a gallon of food and liquid. When your stomach is empty, its tissues fold in on themselves, a bit like a closed accordion. As your stomach fills and expands, the folds gradually disappear.

Your stomach performs two main functions. It continues to process food, breaking it down into smaller pieces, and it stores food, gradually releasing it into your small intestine. Generally, it takes your stomach about four hours to empty after a nutritious meal, and six hours or more if the meal has a lot of fat.

Even before food arrives, stomach juices begin flowing. At the sight, smell and taste of food, your brain begins sending messages along the vagus nerve indicating that food will be coming soon. The vagus nerve carries messages from your brain that control digestion, breathing and circulation. The message it sends to your stomach releases acetylcholine (as-uh-tul-KO-lene). This chemical sets off a chain reaction that starts your stomach muscles contracting and signals your gastric glands to produce digestive juices. Under normal conditions, your stomach produces 2 to 3 quarts of gastric juices every day.

When food arrives from your esophagus, muscles in your upper stomach relax to let it in. The stomach walls, which are lined with three layers of powerful muscles, then begin churning the food, mixing it into smaller and smaller pieces. Gastric juices are released from small glands that line the walls of your stomach. These enzymes help break down food into a thick, creamy fluid called chyme (kime).

Hydrochloric acid is one of many gastric juices. This helpful but corrosive acid could dissolve your stomach if it weren't for the sticky alkaline mucus clinging to your stomach walls. Hydrochloric acid kills harmful bacteria and microorganisms swallowed with the food. Stomach acid also activates pepsin, a protein-digesting enzyme produced by the stomach. Pepsin works mainly on milk. Otherwise, very little chemical digestion and absorption take place in your stomach, except for absorption of aspirin and alcohol. They pass quickly through your stomach lining and into your bloodstream.

Once your food is well mixed, rippling waves of muscles push the stomach contents down toward the pyloric valve leading into the upper portion of your small intestine (duodenum). The pyloric valve, another ring-like sphincter muscle, opens just enough to allow your stomach to release less than an eighth of an ounce of food at a time into the duodenum (doo-o-DEE-num). The rest is held back for more mixing.

Appetite, hunger and feeling full

Appetite is that pleasant feeling that lets you know it's time to eat. Hunger comes later, perhaps when you've gone past your normal mealtime and your body tells you so with unpleasant hunger pangs. Appetite and hunger work together to keep you eating regularly.

Your sensations of appetite and hunger are controlled by a part of your brain called the hypothalamus. A portion of the food you eat is converted into blood sugar (glucose). When your blood sugar level drops, the hypothalamus notices and sends nerve impulses along the vagus nerve to your stomach. These impulses trigger the release of gastric juices, and set in motion the muscle contractions that produce hunger pangs. You may hear your stomach rumbling as juices and air pass through your intestines.

If you aren't able to eat right away, these sensations gradually wear off and you may not feel hungry again for several hours. But later in the day, when it's time for your next meal, you may feel famished.

Once you've eaten, your brain recognizes when you're full. As your stomach fills and stretches to its normal capacity, it signals that your hunger has been satisfied.

The small intestine, pancreas, liver and gallbladder
The small intestine is your body's main digestive organ — a winding passageway that fills much of your abdomen. It's here that the chemical breakdown of food is completed, and where most nutrients are absorbed into your bloodstream. The length of the small intestine varies, but in most adults it's generally about 21 feet long.

Food that's released from your stomach passes into the duodenum, which is about 12 inches long. In this upper portion of your small intestine, breakdown of food continues. Digestive juices are channeled into the duodenum from the following organs.

Pancreas. Your pancreas is a soft, pink gland that lies in your upper abdomen, behind the lower part of your stomach. Shaped a bit like a fish, with a wide head, tapering body and narrow tail, the pancreas is, on average, about 6 inches long and less than 2 inches wide. Among other chemicals, the pancreas produces two important types of secretions. They are:

- The hormones insulin and glucagon, which are secreted into your bloodstream and which help regulate your metabolism, including your level of blood sugar
- Digestive enzymes which are secreted into your bloodstream and which help break down proteins, carbohydrates and fats

Liver. Located on the right side of your body and beneath the lower part of your rib cage, the liver is the largest organ in your body, similar in size to a football. The liver also is one of your most important organs. It's a virtual chemical factory that performs more than 500 functions. They include storing nutrients and filtering and processing chemicals in food. The liver also produces bile, a watery, yellowish-green solution that helps digest fats by breaking large fat globules into smaller ones. This makes digestion easier because it gives fat-digesting enzymes access to more surface area. Like urine, bile also helps eliminate waste products.

Gallbladder. Your gallbladder is part of the system that transports bile, called the biliary tract. It's a small, translucent sac adjacent to your liver that looks green because it stores and concentrates bile produced in your liver. The gallbladder is about 2 to 3 inches long and holds about 2 ounces of bile.

When your body isn't digesting food, bile that's continuously produced by your liver — up to 2 pints a day — drains into bile ducts and then into your gallbladder. There, during storage, the gallbladder absorbs some of the bile's water, which makes up about 95 percent of bile. This reduces the amount of bile and turns the stored bile into a more concentrated, potent solution. When fatty food enters your duodenum, a hormone signals your gallbladder to contract and release its stored bile into the duodenum.

With digestive juices converging from the pancreas, liver and gallbladder — along with others secreted from the walls of the small intestine — digestion reaches its peak. The duodenum, however, can absorb only small amounts of digested food at a time. So its muscular lining contracts and sends the food into the next section of the small intestine.

The second portion of the small intestine, the jejunum (juh-JOO-num), is about 8 feet long. Here is where most digestion is completed. The third and final portion of the small intestine, the ileum (IL-e-um), is about 12 feet long. Its main task is to absorb remaining nutrients through its cell walls. By the time food waste reaches the last portion of the ileum, most vitamins and nutrients have already been absorbed, except for vitamin B-12. Absorption of this essential vitamin occurs in the last few feet of the ileum, called the terminal ileum. Bile acids also are absorbed in the terminal ileum. When bile acids aren't removed from food waste, they pass into the large intestine and may cause diarrhea.

The journey of food through the small intestine generally takes between 30 minutes and three hours, depending on the composition of the meal.

The colon

Also known as the large intestine, the colon stores and removes waste that your body can't digest. Though the colon is shorter than the small intestine — about 5 feet long — its diameter is greater. The colon almost completely frames your small intestine along both sides, top and bottom (see illustration on page 5).

Food enters your colon through yet another muscular (ileocecal) valve that acts as a gateway. This valve at the end of your small intestine opens only one way, so food waste in your colon can't return to the small intestine. By the time food residue reaches the colon, your body has absorbed nearly all of the nutrients it can. What remains are water, electrolytes, such as sodium and chloride, and waste products, such as plant fiber, bacteria, and dead cells shed from the lining of your digestive tract.

During the time when food waste passes through your colon, your body absorbs nearly all of the water from the waste — about 2 to 3 pints each day. The remaining residue, called stool, is usually soft but formed. It's also loaded with bacteria, which are harmless to your body as long as your colon wall remains intact. These bacteria cause certain food products to ferment, producing gas. This gas, called flatus, is mainly an odorless mixture of hydrogen, methane and carbon dioxide. The odors come from certain foods, especially those rich in sulfur, such as garlic and cabbage, and those with sulfur-based preservatives such as bread, beer and potato chips.

Food residue moves through your colon by muscle contraction. Colon contractions separate the waste into small segments. After each meal, considerable movement takes place in the descending colon. During this time, several segments of waste are joined to form stool, which is pushed down into your lower colon and rectum.

As your rectal walls stretch, they signal the need to release stool. The longer you wait to release stool, the more water is absorbed from the waste. This makes stool more compact, hard and difficult to expel (constipation).

Sphincter muscles in your anus serve as a final valve. As your sphincter muscles relax, your rectal walls contract to increase pressure. Sometimes you have to exert pressure from your abdominal muscles, which press on the outside of your colon and rectum. With this coordination of muscles, stool is expelled.

Keeping your tract on track

The health of your digestive system has a lot to do with your lifestyle — the food you eat, the amount of exercise you get, the pace of your day and your level of stress.

Remarkably adaptive, the human digestive system can adjust to a wide variety of foods. It can also tolerate an astonishing amount of stress, as well as abuse from hurried meals. Over time, though, a poor diet and bad eating habits may take their toll. Occasional symptoms, such as heartburn or abdominal pain, may eventually become more frequent and severe.

Not all digestive problems, however, stem from lifestyle. Some conditions are thought to be hereditary or related to an infection. For others, there's no known cause.

In the following chapters, you'll find information to help you take care of your digestive system and help prevent serious problems, along with strategies for identifying and managing conditions that you may already have.

Chapter 2

Recipe for healthy digestion

W hat you put on your plate each day has a great deal to do with good digestion and health. But it's not only what you eat that's important. How much you eat, and the manner in which you eat — relaxed or hurried — also play key roles.

You can't prevent or control all digestive problems simply with lifestyle changes. Some digestive disorders are hereditary, or occur for unknown reasons, and their treatment requires more advanced care. But good lifestyle habits coupled with a good diet can go a long way toward keeping your digestive system healthy.

Eat fiber

Your stomach will accept almost anything you send its way. However, certain foods tend to pass more easily and quickly through your digestive tract and help it function properly. These same foods also form the foundation for a healthy diet.

Plant foods — fruits, vegetables and foods made from whole grains — contain beneficial vitamins, minerals and compounds called phytochemicals that may protect against cancer and heart disease. Plant foods are also excellent sources of fiber, a nutrient that's especially important to digestion.

Fiber comes in two forms — soluble and insoluble. Soluble fiber absorbs up to 15 times its weight in water as it moves through your digestive tract, producing softer stools. It's most abundant in oats, legumes and fruits. Insoluble fiber, found in vegetables and whole grains, gives stool its bulk. Softening and bulking of stool help to prevent constipation, prevent some types of diarrhea, and may help relieve symptoms of irritable bowel syndrome. These actions also decrease pressure in the intestinal tract, reducing your risk of hemorrhoids and diverticular disease, a condition in which pouches form in intestinal walls.

Fiber has other benefits. There's strong evidence that soluble fiber lowers cholesterol and helps protect against cardiovascular disease. It does this by increasing the amount of bile acid — a compound that helps digest fat — excreted in stool. To make more bile acid, your liver removes more cholesterol from your blood. Fiber may also improve diabetes control by slowing digestion, thereby slowing the release of sugar into your bloodstream. However, it's uncertain whether this benefit is from fiber itself, or because high-fiber diets also tend to be low in fat and contain other nutrients that may affect blood sugar control. As for cancer, the benefits of fiber remain unclear. Some studies suggest a high-fiber diet can protect against colon cancer, while others show no protective effect. Despite the lack of conclusive evidence, the scientific consensus is that dietary fiber protects against colon cancer. It's also possible that other components in high-fiber foods, such as phytochemicals, may play a role as protective agents.

Nutrition Facts
Serving Size 6 Wafers (28 g)
Servings Per Container About 10

Amount Per Serving
Calories 130   Calories from Fat 40

	% Daily Value*
Total Fat 4.5 g	7%
Saturated Fat 1 g	4%
Polyunsaturated Fat 0 g	
Monounsaturated Fat 1.5 g	
Cholesterol 0 mg	0%
Sodium 130 mg	5%
Total Carbohydrate 20 g	7%
Dietary Fiber 3 g	13%
Sugars Less than 1 g	
Protein 2 g	

Vitamin A 4%	•	Vitamin C 0%
Calcium 0%	•	Iron 6%
Phosphorus 10%		

Dietary Fiber 3 g   13%

* Percent Daily Values are based on a 2,000-calorie diet. Your daily values may be higher or lower depending on your calorie needs:

	Calories:	2,000	2,500
Total Fat	Less than	65 g	80 g
Sat. Fat	Less than	20 g	25 g
Cholesterol	Less than	300 mg	300 mg
Sodium	Less than	2,400 mg	2,400 mg
Total Carbohydrate		300 g	375 g
Dietary Fiber		25 g	30 g

Packaged foods sold in the United States have a Nutrition Facts label. Nutrition Facts are a quick guide to how a food fits into your eating plan.

Unfortunately, most of us don't get enough fiber. Americans typically consume 10 to 15 grams of fiber daily. Dietary guidelines recommend two to three times that amount. For adults 50 years and younger, the recommendation is 38

Where to find fiber

Depending on your age and sex, aim for 21 to 38 grams of fiber daily from a variety of food sources. To avoid digestive upset and gas that can come from eating too much fiber too quickly, gradually increase the amount you eat over a period of a couple of weeks. Here's the amount of fiber in some common foods.

Breads, cereals and other grain products	Grams		Grams
All-Bran/Extra Fiber, Kellogg's ($\frac{1}{2}$ cup)	13.3	Cheerios, General Mills (1 cup)	3.0
Fiber One, General Mills ($\frac{1}{2}$ cup)	13.0	Rice, brown/cooked (1 cup)	3.5
All-Bran, Kellogg's ($\frac{1}{2}$ cup)	10.0	Pumpernickel bread (1 slice)	2.1
100% Bran, Nabisco ($\frac{1}{3}$ cup)	8.0	Spaghetti, enriched (1 cup cooked)	2.4
Raisin Bran, Post (1 cup)	8.0	Bagel ($3\frac{1}{2}$")	1.6
French bread pizza, Healthy Choice (6 oz.)	7.0	Corn Flakes, Kellogg's (1 cup)	1.1
Shredded Wheat, Quaker (3 biscuits)	7.3	Cracked wheat bread (1 slice)	1.4
Cracklin' Oat Bran, Kellogg's ($\frac{3}{4}$ cup)	5.6	Egg noodles, enriched (1 cup cooked)	1.8
Grape Nuts, Post ($\frac{3}{4}$ cup)	3.0	Oatmeal bread (1 slice)	1.1
Oatmeal, quick/reg./inst. (1 cup cooked)	4.0	Whole-wheat bread (1 slice)	1.9
Bran'ola Original (1 slice)	3.0	White bread (1 slice)	0.6

Fruits			
Avocado, raw/California (1 medium)	8.5	Orange, Valencia (1 medium)	3.0
Raspberries, raw (1 cup)	8.4	Peaches, canned/juice pack (1 cup)	3.2
Dates, dried (10)	6.2	Strawberries, raw (1 cup)	3.4
Prunes (10, dried)	6.0	Banana (1 medium)	2.7
Pears, canned, juice pack (1 cup)	4.0	Applesauce, unsweetened ($\frac{1}{2}$ cup)	1.5
Raisins, seedless ($\frac{2}{3}$ cup)	4.0	Cherries, sweet (10)	1.6
Apple, with skin (1 medium)	3.7	Grapefruit, pink & red ($\frac{1}{2}$ medium)	1.4
Blueberries (1 cup)	3.9	Peach, raw (1 medium)	1.7

Legumes and vegetables (cooked, unless specified)			
Beans, baked, homemade (1 cup)	13.9	Green beans ($\frac{1}{2}$ cup)	2.0
Kidney beans, red, boiled (1 cup)	13.1	Potato, boiled, no skin (1 medium)	2.4
Lima beans ($\frac{1}{2}$ cup)	5.9	Spinach, boiled ($\frac{1}{2}$ cup)	2.2
Chunky Veg. soup, Campbell's (10.75 oz.)	5.0	Squash, acorn ($\frac{1}{2}$ cup cubes, baked)	4.5
Popcorn, air-popped ($3\frac{1}{2}$ cups)	4.2	Cabbage, red ($\frac{1}{2}$ cup, shredded)	1.5
Peas, canned ($\frac{1}{2}$ cup)	3.5	Cauliflower ($\frac{1}{2}$ cup, pieces)	1.3
Sweet potato (1, baked with skin)	3.4	Lettuce, iceberg (1 leaf)	0.3
Broccoli, boiled ($\frac{1}{2}$ cup)	2.3	Onions, raw ($\frac{1}{2}$ cup, chopped)	1.4
Carrots, raw (1 medium)	2.2	Tomato (1 red, raw)	1.4
Corn ($\frac{1}{2}$ cup)	2.3	Celery (1 stalk, raw, $7\frac{1}{2}$" long)	0.7

Cooking ingredients			
Corn bran ($\frac{1}{3}$ cup)	21.4	Oat bran, uncooked ($\frac{1}{3}$ cup)	4.8
Flour, whole-wheat (1 cup)	14.6	Flour, white (1 cup)	3.4
Cornmeal, white/degermed/enr./(1 cup)	10.2	Wheat germ, crude ($\frac{1}{4}$ cup)	3.8
Soy flour, low-fat (1 cup)	9.0	Graham cracker crumbs, Keebler ($\frac{1}{2}$ cup)	1.3

Adapted from: *Bowes & Church's Food Values of Portions Commonly Used*, 17th edition, 1998 grams of fiber a day for men and 25 grams for women. For adults over 50, it's 30 grams for men and 21 grams for women.

The Mayo Clinic Healthy Weight Pyramid (see below) is a dietary guide that can help you increase your fiber intake and promote overall health. It contains recommended types and amounts of foods to eat every day. By emphasizing these foods, you also limit fat. Excess fat slows digestion and can lead to heartburn, bloating and constipation, in addition to increasing your weight, risk of heart disease, diabetes and perhaps colon cancer.

A healthy diet

It's important to eat a well-balanced diet that includes foods from a variety of groups. Try to include the following in your daily diet.

Fruits and vegetables: 8 to 10 servings. Fruits generally have few calories and little or no fat, and they contain beneficial fiber, vitamins, minerals and phytochemicals. Fresh fruits are generally higher in fiber than are canned fruits. Dried fruits are high in fiber, but they're also higher in calories.

Vegetables are naturally low in calories and most are fat-free.

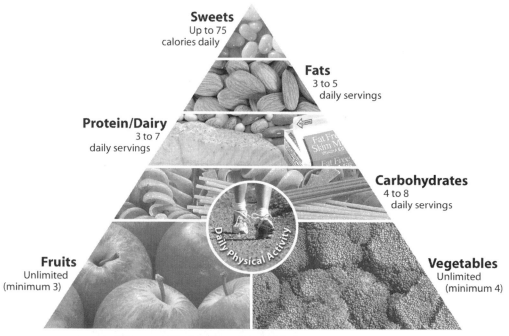

Mayo Clinic Healthy Weight Pyramid
See your doctor before you begin any healthy weight plan.

They provide fiber, vitamins, minerals and phytochemicals.

Carbohydrates: 4 to 8 servings. These include grains — cereals, breads, rice and pasta — rich in energy-filled complex carbohydrates and important nutrients.

Along with vegetables and fruits, carbohydrates form the foundation of a healthy diet. Select whole grains when possible, because they contain more fiber than do refined varieties.

Protein/Dairy: 3 to 7 servings. This group includes foods from both plant and animal sources. Plant-based foods rich in protein include legumes such as beans, peas and lentils. They're low in fat and cholesterol-free. They're also excellent sources of fiber. Animal-based foods rich in protein include fish and seafood, poultry, meat and eggs. These foods are also sources of B vitamins, iron and zinc. However, because even lean varieties contain fat and cholesterol,

Sizing up a serving

The number of servings recommended for each food group may sound like a lot of food, but serving sizes may be smaller than you think. Here are some examples of what counts as one serving.

Food	Serving examples
Grains	1 slice whole-wheat bread $\frac{1}{2}$ bagel or English muffin $\frac{1}{2}$ cup (3 oz./84 g) cooked cereal, rice or pasta $\frac{1}{2}$ to 1 cup (1 oz./28 g) ready-to-eat cereal
Fruits and vegetables	$\frac{3}{4}$ cup (6 fl. oz./180 mL) 100 percent fruit juice 1 medium orange, apple, banana or pear 1 cup (2 oz./56 g) raw leafy vegetables $\frac{1}{2}$ cup (3 oz./ 84 g) cooked or chopped raw vegetables 1 medium potato
Dairy products	1 cup (8 fl. oz./240 mL) low-fat or fat-free milk or yogurt $1\frac{1}{2}$ oz. (42 g) natural cheese, such as cheddar 2 oz. (56 g) processed cheese, such as American $\frac{1}{2}$ cup (4 oz./125 g) low-fat or fat-free cottage cheese
Poultry, fish, meat	2-3 oz. (56-84 g) cooked skinless poultry, fish or lean meat
Legumes	$\frac{1}{2}$ cup ($3\frac{1}{2}$oz./98 g) cooked legumes (beans, dried peas or lentils)

try to limit your total intake of animal-based protein to 6 ounces or less a day.

Dairy products high in protein include milk, yogurt and cheese, which are also outstanding sources of calcium and vitamin D, which help your body absorb calcium. Some dairy products are high in fat and cholesterol, so low-fat or fat-free products are your best choices.

Fats, sweets and alcohol: Sparingly. Alcohol, fats and sugars provide calories but no nutrients. To cut fat in your diet, reduce the amount of butter, margarine and oils that you use in cooking. Also limit sweets, such as candy, desserts and sugar-sweetened soft drinks.

Drink plenty of fluids

Fluids promote healthy digestion by lubricating food waste so that it passes more easily through your digestive tract. Fluids also soften stool, helping to prevent constipation. In addition, they help dissolve vitamins, minerals and other nutrients, making them easier for your tissues to absorb.

Water is generally the best way in which to get fluid. Milk, juices and other beverages are about 90 percent water, so they also can help meet your daily fluid needs (see "How much is enough?"). Caffeinated beverages and alcohol don't count. In some people, they act as diuretics, increasing urination and fluid loss. Caffeine and alcohol may also contribute to heartburn and indigestion.

In the morning, a warm beverage may be preferable to a cold one, especially if you're bothered by constipation. About 30 minutes after drinking warm liquid, your body may have a natural urge to pass stool. Drinking a caffeinated beverage may also stimulate a bowel movement.

How much is enough?

To determine the amount of fluid your body needs, divide your weight (in pounds) in half. The answer is the approximate amount of fluid (in ounces) recommended daily. For most people, the figure equates to at least eight 8-ounce glasses.

Practice good eating habits

Just as important as what you eat is the manner in which you eat. Poor digestion may simply be due to bad habits.

Eat moderate proportions

Your body is able to produce only a certain volume of digestive juices. Large meals put increased demands on digestion. Large amounts of food can also increase the amount of waste moving through your digestive tract, which in turn may lead to bloating. Moderate portions, on the other hand, are digested more comfortably. Overeating also can lead to overweight and obesity.

Eat at regular times

Your digestive organs operate best when you follow a regular schedule — breakfast, lunch and dinner. Skipping meals can lead to excessive hunger, which often results in overeating. People who eat whenever they feel like it or have time also tend to eat less nutritious foods than those who eat three meals a day. With a regular schedule, your digestive system also has time to rest between meals.

Relax while you eat

This is as important as eating at set times. When you're relaxed, you tend to chew your food more completely, gastric and intestinal juices flow more freely, and digestive muscles contract and relax normally. When you eat too fast, you don't chew food thoroughly and often swallow air, causing heartburn or bloating and gas. Eating while you feel stressed interferes with normal functioning of your intestines, and can result in stomach upset, bloating, constipation or diarrhea.

Maintain a healthy weight

Digestive problems can occur no matter what your weight. But heartburn, bloating and constipation tend to be more common in people who are overweight, perhaps because they tend to exercise less and eat more fat and less fiber. Maintaining a healthy weight can often help prevent or reduce these problems.

Is your weight healthy?

Three do-it-yourself evaluations can tell you whether your weight is healthy or whether you could benefit from weight loss.

Body mass index. Body mass index (BMI) is a formula that considers your weight and your height in determining whether you have a healthy or unhealthy percentage of body fat. Generally, the higher your BMI, the greater is your risk of diabetes, high blood pressure, cardiovascular disease and cancer.

To determine your body mass index, locate your height on the chart in "What's your BMI?" on page 21 and follow it across until you reach the weight nearest yours. Look at the top of the column for the BMI rating. (If your weight is less than the weight nearest yours, your BMI may be slightly less. If your weight is greater than the weight nearest yours, your BMI may be slightly greater.) A BMI of 19 to 24.9 is considered healthy. A BMI of 25 to 29.9 signifies overweight, and a BMI of 30 or more indicates obesity. If your BMI is less than 18.5, you're underweight, which may also put you at increased risk.

Waist circumference. This measurement indicates where most of your body fat is located. People who carry most of their weight around their waists sometimes are referred to as apple shaped. Those who carry most of their weight below the waist, around their hips and thighs, may be referred to as pear shaped.

Generally, it's better to have a pear shape than an apple shape. That's because excess fat around your abdomen is generally associated with a greater risk of heart attack and other weight-related diseases.

To determine whether you're carrying too much weight around your abdomen, measure your waist circumference just above your hipbones, usually at the level of your navel. A measurement of more than 40 inches (102 centimeters) in men and 35 inches (89 centimeters) in women signifies increased health risks, especially if you have a BMI of 25 or higher.

Personal and family history. An evaluation of your medical history, along with that of your family, is also important in determining whether your weight is healthy. Ask yourself these questions:

What's your BMI?

	Normal		Overweight					Obese				
BMI	19	24	25	26	27	28	29	30	35	40	45	50
Height						Weight in pounds						
4'10"	91	115	119	124	129	134	138	143	167	191	215	239
4'11"	94	119	124	128	133	138	143	148	173	198	222	247
5'0"	97	123	128	133	138	143	148	153	179	204	230	255
5'1"	100	127	132	137	143	148	153	158	185	211	238	264
5'2"	104	131	136	142	147	153	158	164	191	218	246	273
5'3"	107	135	141	146	152	158	163	169	197	225	254	282
5'4"	110	140	145	151	157	163	169	174	204	232	262	291
5'5"	114	144	150	156	162	168	174	180	210	240	270	300
5'6"	118	148	155	161	167	173	179	186	216	247	278	309
5'7"	121	153	159	166	172	178	185	191	223	255	287	319
5'8"	125	158	164	171	177	184	190	197	230	262	295	328
5'9"	128	162	169	176	182	189	196	203	236	270	304	338
5'10"	132	167	174	181	188	195	202	209	243	278	313	348
5'11"	136	172	179	186	193	200	208	215	250	286	322	358
6'0"	140	177	184	191	199	206	213	221	258	294	331	368
6'1"	144	182	189	197	204	212	219	227	265	302	340	378
6'2"	148	186	194	202	210	218	225	233	272	311	350	389
6'3"	152	192	200	208	216	224	232	240	279	319	359	399
6'4"	156	197	205	213	221	230	238	246	287	328	369	410

Source: National Institutes of Health (NIH), 1998

- Do you have a health condition, such as gastroesophageal reflux disease (GERD), that would benefit from weight loss?
- Do you have a family history of a weight-related illness, such as diabetes, high blood pressure, or colon or breast cancer?
- Have you gained considerable weight since high school? Weight gain in adulthood is associated with increased health risks.
- Do you smoke cigarettes, have more than two alcoholic drinks a day or live with considerable stress? In combination with these behaviors, excess weight can have greater health implications.

Do you need to lose weight?

If your BMI shows that you aren't overweight and you're not carrying too much weight around your abdomen, there's probably no health advantage to changing your weight. Your weight is healthy.

If your BMI is between 25 and 29.9, your waist circumference exceeds healthy guidelines, or you answered yes to at least one personal and family health question, you might benefit from losing a few pounds. Discuss your weight with your doctor during your next checkup.

If your BMI is 30 or more, losing weight is recommended to improve your overall health and energy level and to help reduce your risk of illness.

If you need to lose weight

The best way to lose weight safely, and keep it off, is through lifestyle changes. Many products and programs promise to help you shed pounds, but they aren't always safe or effective. Too many people eventually gain back the weight they lost.

Here are some steps that can help you be successful.

Make a commitment. You must be motivated to lose weight because it's what you want, not what someone else wants you to do. Only you can help yourself lose weight. However, that doesn't mean that you have to act alone. Your doctor, a registered dietitian, or other health care professional can help you develop a plan to lose weight.

Think positively. Don't dwell on what you're giving up to lose weight. Instead, concentrate on what you're gaining. Instead of thinking, "I really miss eating a doughnut for breakfast," tell yourself, "I feel a lot better when I eat whole-wheat toast and cereal in the morning."

Get your priorities straight. Timing is crucial. Don't try to lose weight while you're distracted by other problems. It takes a lot of mental and physical energy to change habits. If you're having family or financial problems, or a friend or family member is ill, it may not be the best time to try to lose weight.

Set a realistic goal. Don't aim for an unrealistic weight that meets social ideals of thinness. Instead, try for a comfortable weight that you maintained as a young adult. If you've always been overweight, aim for a weight that will improve your digestive symptoms and your energy level. Even modest weight loss — about 10 percent of your weight — can have significant health benefits.

Accept the fact that healthy weight loss is slow and steady. A good weight-loss plan generally involves losing no more than 1/2 to 2 pounds a week. Set weekly or monthly goals that allow you to keep track of your successes.

Know your habits. Ask yourself if you tend to eat when you're bored, angry, tired, anxious, depressed or feeling pressured. If you do, try these solutions:

- Before eating anything, ask yourself if you really want it.
- Do something to distract yourself from your desire to eat, such as telephoning a friend or running an errand.
- If you're feeling stressed or angry, direct that energy constructively. Instead of eating, take a brisk walk.

Don't starve yourself. Liquid meals, diet pills and special food combinations aren't the answer to long-term weight control and better health. The best way to lose weight is to eat more nutritious foods — whole grains, fruits and vegetables — and fewer foods that contain fat and sugar.

Most people try to lose weight by eating only 1,000 to 1,500 calories a day. Cutting calories to fewer than 1,200 if you're a woman or 1,400 if you're a man doesn't provide enough food to keep you satisfied, and you get hungry before your next meal. Eating fewer than 1,200 calories makes it difficult to get adequate amounts of certain nutrients. It also promotes temporary loss of fluids and a loss of healthy muscle, instead of permanent loss of fat.

Remain committed. Don't let occasional setbacks — and there will be some — weaken your commitment to lose weight. If you find yourself falling back into an old, bad habit, use the strategies you followed in breaking that habit in the first place. It's not enough to eat nutritious foods and exercise for a few weeks, or even several months. You have to incorporate these new, beneficial behaviors into your life.

Weight-loss medications and surgery. Prescription medications for weight loss are appropriate for moderately overweight and obese people who have health complications related to weight and who are enrolled in a weight management program that emphasizes healthy nutrition and physical activity. Drugs can be a tool to help make changes in diet, not the solution to the problem.

Generally, surgery for weight loss is reserved for people who are severely obese and who have health problems as a result. Surgery may be considered if you have a BMI above 40 or if you have weight-related health problems.

Increase your activity level. Dieting alone will help you lose weight. But by incorporating exercise into your daily routine, you can increase your weight loss. Exercise is the most important factor related to long-term healthy weight management.

Get regular exercise

Aerobic exercise — exercise that increases your breathing and heart rate — is the most beneficial for healthy digestion. In addition to improving heart and lung health, aerobic exercise stimulates the activity of intestinal muscles, helping to move food and waste through your intestines. Aerobic exercise also promotes weight loss, builds stamina and helps to strengthen your immune system.

Try to do 30 to 60 minutes of aerobic activity most, if not all, days of the week. Walking is the most common aerobic activity because it's easy, convenient and inexpensive. All you need is a good pair of walking shoes. Other aerobic exercises include:

Borg Ratings of Perceived Exertion Scale

Perceived exertion refers to the total amount of effort, physical stress and fatigue you experience during a physical activity. For the activity to be most beneficial, try to aim for a rating of 13 — somewhat hard.

6 No exertion at all	11 Light	16
7 Extremely light	12	17 Very hard
8	13 Somewhat hard	18
9 Very light	14	19 Extremely hard
10	15 Hard (heavy)	20 Maximal exertion

© Gunnar Borg 1998

- Bicycling
- Golfing (walking, not riding)
- Volleyball
- Hiking
- Skiing
- Tennis

- Basketball
- Social dancing
- Aerobic dancing
- Jogging
- Running
- Swimming

A total fitness program

Aerobic exercise is just one component of a total fitness program. Stretching and strengthening exercises also are important for good health. Stretching before and after aerobic activity increases the range to which you can bend and stretch your joints, muscles and ligaments. Stretching also helps prevent joint pain and injury.

Strengthening exercises, such as lifting weights and using resistance machines, can build stronger muscles that in turn

Before you get started

It's often a good idea to talk with your doctor before starting an exercise program. If you have a health problem or you're at risk of heart disease, you may need to take some precautions while you exercise.

It's essential that you see your doctor if you:
- Are unsure of your health status
- Have experienced chest discomfort, shortness of breath or dizziness during or right after exercise or strenuous activity
- Are a man age 40 years or older, or a woman age 50 years or older, and haven't had a recent physical examination
- Have a blood pressure of 140/90 millimeters of mercury or higher
- Have diabetes, heart, lung or kidney disease, or are obese
- Have a family history of heart-related problems before age 55
- Are taking medication for diabetes, high blood pressure, heart problems or another medical condition
- Have bone or joint problems that could be made worse by some forms of physical activity

improve posture, balance and coordination. Strength training also promotes healthy bones and increases your rate of metabolism, which can help keep your weight in check.

Remember that you don't have to get in all your exercise at one time. Doing 20 minutes of walking during the morning, 15 minutes of lawn mowing in the afternoon and perhaps 25 minutes of bicycling in the evening all count toward keeping fit.

Control stress

Digestive troubles can occur for reasons other than a poor diet or lack of exercise. Your digestive tract is long and complex, and many lifestyle components can influence how well it functions. One of the most important is stress.

Everyone experiences stress. What's important is to recognize when you're feeling stressed, and to take steps to relieve your tension with exercise or relaxation techniques. Left untreated, stress can adversely affect digestion.

When you're stressed, your body reacts as if you're in danger. It pumps extra blood to your muscles so that you have more energy to fight off an attack or run away. This leaves less blood volume to support digestion. Your digestive muscles exert less effort, compounds (enzymes) that aid digestion are secreted in smaller amounts, and passage of food and waste through your digestive tract shifts into low gear. This can produce symptoms such as heartburn, bloating and constipation.

Sometimes stress does the opposite. It speeds passage of food through your intestines, causing abdominal pain and diarrhea. Stress also may worsen symptoms of conditions such as ulcers, irritable bowel syndrome and ulcerative colitis.

Limit alcohol

There's increasing evidence that some alcoholic beverages may have beneficial health effects, especially in reducing your risk of heart disease. But it's best to limit alcohol to a moderate amount — no more than one drink a day if you're a woman or two drinks a day if you're a man, and just one drink a day regardless of your sex if you're over 65. A drink is defined as 12 ounces of beer, 5 ounces of wine, or 1.5 ounces of 80-proof distilled spirits.

Too much alcohol — anything above a moderate amount — can lead to many serious problems, including some digestive disorders. Alcohol can inflame your stomach lining and relax your lower esophageal sphincter, the valve that prevents stomach acid from backing up into your esophagus. These actions can cause bleeding or heartburn. Alcohol can aggravate symptoms such as diarrhea or nausea. Excessive alcohol is a leading cause of liver and pancreatic disease. When combined with tobacco, alcohol greatly increases your risk of mouth and esophageal cancers.

Avoid tobacco

If you chew or smoke tobacco, you may be more likely to experience heartburn. That's because nicotine in tobacco may increase stomach acid production and decrease production of sodium bicarbonate, a fluid that neutralizes stomach acid. Air swallowed during smoking can produce belching or bloating from gas. In addition, smoking puts you at increased risk of peptic ulcers and cancers of the mouth, throat and esophagus.

Use medications cautiously

Almost all medications affect digestion in one way or another. Often the effects are mild and go unnoticed, but some drugs can produce noticeable signs and symptoms, especially if you take them regularly. For example, narcotics taken to relieve pain can produce constipation, medications taken for high blood pressure can cause diarrhea or constipation, and antibiotics taken to fight infection can cause nausea or diarrhea.

Some of the most potentially damaging medications, however, are nonsteroidal anti-inflammatory drugs (NSAIDs). These medications include the over-the-counter drugs aspirin, ibuprofen (Advil, Motrin, others), naproxen (Aleve) and ketoprofen (Orudis ICT). When taken occasionally and as directed, the drugs are generally safe.

When taken regularly, or if you take more than the recommended amount, they may cause nausea, stomach pain, stomach bleeding or ulcers. That's because NSAIDs inhibit production of an enzyme called cyclooxygenase (COX). This enzyme produces hormone-like substances called prostaglandins that trigger inflammation and pain. However, prostaglandins also have a beneficial effect. They help protect your stomach lining against harmful acid.

If you take an NSAID regularly, talk with your doctor about ways to limit the drug's side effects, including taking the medication with food.

The newer class of medications called COX-2 inhibitors are generally less damaging to your digestive system than are NSAIDs. Unlike NSAIDs, these medications interfere mainly with the production of prostaglandins associated with inflammation and pain, and less with those involved in digestion. Several studies have shown COX-2 inhibitors relieve joint pain with fewer side effects than traditional NSAIDs. However, more recent studies have found an increased risk of cardiovascular problems, including heart attack and stroke, in some people who used COX-2 inhibitors long-term. Other serious but rare side effects may include stomach or intestinal bleeding, kidney or liver problems and allergic reactions. Because COX-2 inhibitors have been available for a relatively short time, all of their possible long-term effects aren't yet known.

Chapter 3

Gut feelings

You know the feeling. You've had it before, and you'll most likely have it again. It may be that uneasy sense of nausea headed your way, or diarrhea urging you on to the nearest bathroom. Perhaps it's that all too familiar sear of heartburn after a large meal.

Digestive symptoms such as these are common. Almost everyone experiences them from time to time. Usually, the symptoms aren't anything to worry about. After a few hours, they gradually ease and disappear.

It's when digestive symptoms persist or worsen that they may indicate a more serious illness that needs medical attention. The most common digestive complaints — and reasons people see a doctor — include:

- Difficulty swallowing
- Chest pain and heartburn
- Belching, bloating and intestinal gas
- Indigestion
- Nausea and vomiting
- Abdominal pain
- Diarrhea or constipation
- Bleeding
- Weight loss

If you're bothered by a specific sign or symptom but you're unsure of the cause, this chapter may help you better understand what may — or may not — be producing it. It's still important, however, that you see your doctor for a thorough examination.

Difficulty swallowing

Most people take swallowing for granted. They take a bite of food, chew, swallow and don't give it a second thought. But for other people, difficulty swallowing can be a daily problem.

If you get the feeling when you swallow that food is sticking in your throat or chest, you may have dysphagia (dis-FA-je-uh). The term comes from the Greek words *dys* (difficult) and *phagia* (to eat). Dysphagia can occur in two locations.

Pharynx

The pharynx is at the back of the throat and leads into your esophagus. If you have pharyngeal dysphagia, you have trouble moving food from your mouth and throat into your upper esophagus. The problem generally stems from weakened throat muscles because of a stroke or a neuromuscular disorder, such as muscular dystrophy or Parkinson's disease. Other signs and symptoms may include choking or coughing while swallowing, regurgitating fluid (or sometimes food) through the nose, a weak voice and weight loss.

Esophagus

Esophageal dysphagia is more common. It refers to the sensation of food sticking or getting hung up in your esophagus. The sensation is often accompanied by pressure or pain in your chest. Other signs and symptoms may include:

- Painful swallowing
- Belching
- Persistent cough
- Sore throat
- Gurgling sounds
- Bad breath

There are many reasons for esophageal dysphagia. One of the most common is a narrowing of the lower esophagus from formation of scar tissue. The scar tissue is caused by stomach acid backing up into the esophagus and inflaming its tissues (gastroesophageal reflux disease, or GERD).

Tumors (noncancerous or cancerous), radiation burns from cancer treatment, or a band of tissue that narrows the lower esophagus (Schatzki's ring) also can cause dysphagia. In addition, muscles that line your esophagus and propel food to your stomach can weaken with age, making it more difficult for you to swallow. Diseases that affect movement of food through the esophagus, such as achalasia or scleroderma, do so by weakening esophageal muscles.

One other possible cause of dysphagia is a diverticulum, a small pouch that can form in the back of your pharynx, just above the esophagus. Food particles may enter the pouch, where they may be regurgitated, producing gurgling sounds and bad breath. Regurgitated particles also may travel into your lungs, causing a cough and sometimes difficult breathing.

An occasional episode of swallowing difficulty typically isn't a serious problem, and may simply stem from not chewing your food well enough or eating too fast. But if you frequently have trouble swallowing, or your symptoms are severe, see your doctor.

Treating dysphagia

Treatment of dysphagia depends on its cause.

Physical therapy. If your swallowing difficulty is a result of weakened muscles, a physical therapist may assist you with techniques to help you swallow better.

Drug therapy. For dysphagia stemming from GERD, prescription medications are often effective in preventing reflux of stomach acid into the esophagus. For dysphagia associated with spasm of your esophageal muscles, muscle-relaxing drugs can help control the spasms.

Tissue stretching. If your esophagus is narrowed, causing food to hang up, your doctor may insert a slender, flexible tube (endoscope) down your esophagus, and thread through the tube a device to stretch (dilate) narrowed tissues. Often, the device is a deflated balloon that's placed in the narrowing and then inflated to widen the passageway.

Surgery. In case of a tumor or a diverticulum, surgery is often necessary.

Modified diet. Sometimes it's necessary to modify the consistency of your diet until the cause of the problem is diagnosed and treated. Depending on the type and extent of your dysphagia, you may need to limit your diet to soft, pureed or liquid foods.

To learn more

For additional information on conditions that may cause swallowing difficulty see these chapters.

- Chapter 5: Gastroesophageal reflux disease (GERD)
- Chapter 14: Cancer

Chest pain and heartburn

Pain in your chest can occur for a number of reasons. It could be a warning sign of a heart attack. The pain may stem from lack of oxygen to your heart muscle during exertion (angina pectoris), a lung condition, or inflammation of the cartilage in your rib cage.

Many times, though, chest pain isn't heart- or lung-related. Rather, it stems from a digestive problem. Muscle spasms in your esophagus can produce chest pain. The pain associated with gallbladder inflammation (a gallbladder attack) also can spread to the chest. The most common type of digestive-related chest pain, however, is pain that's commonly known as heartburn.

Heartburn is a term to describe the burning sensation in your chest that may start in your upper abdomen and radiate all the way up into your neck. Heartburn isn't a disease. Rather, it's a symptom. At times, especially when you're lying down, heartburn can be associated with a sour taste in your mouth from stomach acid that backs up into your esophagus and mouth.

Normally, digestive acid remains in your stomach, kept there by the lower esophageal sphincter. This ring of muscle functions as a valve, which opens only when you swallow. But sometimes the valve relaxes or weakens, allowing stomach acid to regurgitate into your esophagus, producing a burning sensation. Many infants are born with an immature sphincter, which is why they often spit up milk or food. By age 1, the valve is more fully developed and reflux becomes less common.

Among adults, heartburn can occur for many reasons. Being overweight, overeating, or lying down too soon after a meal puts pressure on the sphincter muscle, causing it to open slightly. Through the small opening, stomach acid flows into the esophagus. Too much alcohol or caffeine and certain foods also can relax the sphincter or increase production of stomach acid.

Occasional bouts of heartburn are common, and often they stem from overeating, drinking too much alcohol or going to bed with a full stomach. However, if you have heartburn several times a week or you take antacids daily, see your doctor. Your heartburn may be a symptom of a more serious condition, such as GERD. If your heartburn seems worse or different from normal — especially if it's accompanied by radiating pain in an arm — seek medical help immediately. Instead of heartburn, your pain may be a warning of a heart attack.

To learn more
For additional information on conditions that may produce heartburn or chest pain see these chapters.
- Chapter 5: Gastroesophageal reflux disease (GERD)
- Chapter 11: Gallstones

Belching, bloating and intestinal gas

Buildup of air and gas in your digestive tract is a natural part of the digestive process. When you swallow food, you often swallow air with it. Too much air in your digestive tract can lead to belching, bloating or passage of gas from your rectum (flatulence). Another source of gas formation is food residue in your colon. Bacteria naturally present in your colon begin to ferment the undigested food particles, producing gas and bloating.

It's natural to pass gas or to experience occasional discomfort from gas or air buildup. Excessive belching, bloating or gas, however, can be a persistent source of embarrassment and discomfort.

Belching
Belching, or burping, is your body's way of expelling excess air that you swallow while eating or drinking. This can happen from eating too fast, talking while you eat or drinking carbonated beverages.

When you belch, air from your stomach is forced into your esophagus and out of your mouth. Some people who belch repeatedly — even when they're not eating or drinking — swallow air as a nervous habit. Belching also can result from reflux of acid from your stomach into your esophagus. To clear the material, you may swallow frequently, which leads to more intake of air and further belching.

To reduce belching, you want to swallow less air. These suggestions can help.

Eat and drink slowly. The slower you eat and drink, the less air you swallow.

Cut down on carbonated drinks and beer. They contain air.

Avoid gum and hard candy. When you suck on hard candy or chew gum, you swallow more often than normal. Part of what you're swallowing is air.

Don't use a straw. You swallow more air this way than you do when you drink from a glass.

Don't smoke. When you inhale smoke, you also inhale and swallow air.

Check your dentures. Loosefitting dentures can cause you to swallow excess air while you drink or eat.

If these steps don't improve your symptoms, see your doctor to rule out more serious conditions associated with belching, such as GERD or gastritis.

Bloating

Bloating is the common term for gas buildup in your stomach and intestines. Many times, bloating is accompanied by abdominal pain that may be either mild and dull or sharp and intense.

Most often, bloating results from eating a lot of fatty foods. Fat delays stomach emptying and can increase the sensation of fullness. In some instances, bloating may be related to an intestinal abnormality, such as celiac disease or lactose (milk sugar) intolerance, conditions in which your intestines aren't able to absorb certain food components (see "Living with lactose intolerance" on page 36, and Chapter 9: "Celiac disease"). Bloating can result from a gastrointestinal infection or blockage. It also may accompany conditions such as irritable bowel syndrome and may be related to stress or anxiety. Bloating may be associated with delayed stomach emptying (gastroparesis), a problem for some people with diabetes. Another cause of bloating can be fructose intolerance — the inability to properly digest the simple sugar found in fruit and many processed foods. It may also result simply from swallowing air while eating too fast. Passing gas or having a bowel movement may relieve the discomfort.

Intestinal gas (flatus)

Occasionally, some of the air that you swallow will make it all the way into your colon, and is expelled through your anus instead of your mouth. Gas also can form when your intestines have difficulty breaking down certain components in foods, including the sugars in milk products and fruit. Most often, though, gas results from fermentation of undigested food, such as plant fiber, in your colon. Intestinal (colonic) gas is composed mainly of five odorless substances — oxygen, nitrogen, hydrogen, carbon dioxide and methane. Foul smells that may accompany passage of gas come from other gases containing sulfur that are produced by decomposing food particles in the colon. Constipation also can lead to intestinal gas. The longer food waste remains in your colon, the more time it has to ferment.

The following practices can help reduce gas.

Limit foods that produce gas. Common gas-producers include:

- Apples
- Bananas
- Beans
- Bran cereals
- Broccoli
- Brussels sprouts
- Cabbage
- Cauliflower
- Cucumbers
- Melons
- Onions
- Peas
- Prunes
- Radishes
- Raisins

Eating fewer fatty foods, such as fried meats, cream sauces, gravies and rich pastries also may help. Fatty foods often slow digestion, giving food more time to ferment. The artificial sweeteners sorbitol and mannitol, found in dietetic candies and sugar-free gums, also can produce gas.

Living with lactose intolerance

You love dairy products, but they don't love you. Shortly after a bowl of ice cream or a serving of cheesy lasagna, you experience cramps, bloating, gas and diarrhea — signs and symptoms that come from a reduced ability to digest milk sugar (lactose), called lactose (LAK-tose) intolerance.

To digest lactose, you need the enzyme lactase (LAK-tase). Babies are born with large amounts of lactase. But as you grow older, your body often produces less lactase. Adults whose intestines produce very little, if any, lactase are lactase deficient and can't digest any foods containing lactose. Between 30 million and 50 million Americans are lactose intolerant.

Tolerance to lactose varies. Most people can handle the amount of lactose in half a cup of milk, and they don't have a problem consuming small amounts of dairy products throughout the day. Symptoms occur when they consume several dairy products at one time, or they eat a large portion of a product that contains lactose. People with more severe intolerance aren't able to eat any dairy products without experiencing distressing symptoms.

To reduce symptoms of lactose intolerance, avoid these high-lactose foods or eat them in small amounts.

- Cheese spreads
- Chip dip or potato topping
- Cottage cheese
- Dry milk
- Evaporated milk
- Half-and-half
- Ice cream or ice milk
- Milk
- Ricotta cheese
- Sour cream
- Sweetened condensed milk
- White sauces

Yogurt is a good food choice because bacteria in yogurt digest much of the lactose in the product. Look for yogurt with active yeast cultures. Other foods that are lower in lactose include aged cheeses, butter, margarine and sherbet. Nondairy creamers are lactose-free.

Tablets or drops sold in stores under brand names such as Lactaid contain the enzyme lactase and can often prevent or relieve symptoms of lactose intolerance. Some milk sold in grocery stores also contains lactase.

It's important, however, that you not remove nutritious foods, such as vegetables and fruits, from your diet completely just because they may cause gas. A registered dietitian can discuss food choices with you to ensure that you still eat a healthy diet, while reducing gas. You might also try over-the-counter products such as Beano (a food enzyme), which reduces gas formation, or products containing simethicone, intended to relieve gas.

Add fiber gradually. High-fiber foods are good for digestion and your health. But eating too much fiber too quickly can cause gas. Increase fiber in your diet gradually over a period of several weeks. A dietitian can give you advice on which high-fiber foods are less likely to produce gas.

Exercise regularly. Regular exercise reduces intestinal gas by helping to prevent constipation. It can also help get rid of bloating.

Drink plenty of water. Like exercise, water helps to prevent constipation thereby reducing gas.

To learn more
For additional information on conditions that may produce belching, bloating or gas, see these chapters.
- Chapter 5: Gastroesophageal reflux disease (GERD)
- Chapter 7: Irritable bowel syndrome
- Chapter 9: Celiac disease

Indigestion

People often visit the doctor for what they call indigestion. The term is used to describe a number of signs and symptoms — abdominal discomfort, nausea, heartburn, and bloating accompanied by belching. Most commonly, though, people associate indigestion with stomach pain (dyspepsia). Common causes include:
- Peptic ulcers
- Stomach inflammation (gastritis) from medications, alcohol or an infection
- Nonulcer dyspepsia
Nonulcer dyspepsia is a condition in which people experience

symptoms that resemble those of an ulcer, but in which an ulcer doesn't exist.

Less commonly, stomach pain or discomfort can be a symptom of other digestive disorders, such as gallbladder inflammation or pancreatic disease.

An occasional episode of dyspepsia generally isn't anything to worry about, and may even be related to hunger pangs. But if you're having persistent, recurrent or severe pain or discomfort, see your doctor.

To learn more

For additional information on conditions that may produce stomach pain or discomfort, see these chapters.
- Chapter 6: Ulcers and stomach pain
- Chapter 11: Gallstones
- Chapter 12: Pancreatitis

Nausea and vomiting

Most people experience an occasional bout of nausea and vomiting. Often, the culprit is gastroenteritis (gas-tro-en-tur-I-tis), an inflammation of the lining of the stomach and intestines. The most common causes of gastroenteritis are a viral infection or bacteria from spoiled food. Nausea and vomiting also can result from high levels of toxins in your blood, including alcohol or drugs, or from increased levels of hormones produced during pregnancy or periods of intense stress.

Nausea and vomiting may also occur because of increased pressure inside the skull due to fluid accumulation or a tumor. An intense headache or an inner-ear disturbance, including motion sickness, also can lead to nausea and vomiting.

Nausea and vomiting generally aren't signs and symptoms of serious disease unless they persist or are accompanied by pain. If the vomit looks like coffee grounds (partially digested blood) or it contains blood, see your doctor promptly. Depending on other signs and symptoms, you could have a digestive condition such as an ulcer, gallstones, pancreatitis, liver disease or an obstruction in your intestines.

Self-care

For infrequent nausea and vomiting due to a virus or bacteria, the following may help limit your discomfort and prevent dehydration:

- Stop eating and drinking for a few hours until your stomach has settled.
- Avoid food odors. Eat cold foods or those that don't require cooking.
- When you begin to feel better, suck on ice chips or take small sips of water, weak tea, clear soft drinks, noncaffeinated sports drinks, or broth. Sip beverages often to prevent dehydration.
- Gradually add easily digested foods such as gelatin, crackers and dry toast. Once you can tolerate these, try mild-flavored, nonfatty foods such as cereal, rice and fruits.
- For several days avoid fatty or spicy foods, caffeine, alcohol, and aspirin or other nonsteroidal anti-inflammatory drugs.

To learn more

For additional information on conditions that may produce nausea and vomiting, see these chapters.

- Chapter 6: Ulcers and stomach pain
- Chapter 11: Gallstones
- Chapter 12: Pancreatitis
- Chapter 13: Liver disease

Abdominal pain

Abdominal pain can occur alone, or it may accompany other digestive symptoms. Occasional episodes of pain often stem from overeating or eating too much of the wrong foods — fatty foods, gas-producing foods or, for people with lactose intolerance, dairy products. Usually the pain goes away within a few hours. In case of a viral or bacterial infection, it may linger for one or two days.

Abdominal pain that's recurrent, persists, is severe or is accompanied by other signs and symptoms may signal a potentially serious condition. The location of the pain may help your doctor narrow the list of possible causes. However, sometimes the location can be misleading.

Navel area. Pain near your navel often is related to a small intestine disorder or an inflammation of your appendix (appendicitis). The appendix is a worm-shaped pouch that projects out from your colon. It can become clogged with food waste that can cause it to inflame, swell and fill with pus. Without treatment, an infected appendix can burst and cause a serious infection (peritonitis). In addition to pain around your navel and later in your lower right abdomen, other signs and symptoms of appendicitis may include nausea, vomiting, loss of appetite, a low-grade fever, and the urge to pass gas or have a bowel movement.

Above the navel. Directly above the navel is the epigastric area. This is where you might expect to feel pain associated with stomach disorders. Persistent pain in this area also may signal a problem with your upper small intestine (duodenum), pancreas or gallbladder.

Below the navel. Pain below the navel and spreading to either side may signify a colon disorder. Other common causes of pain in this area are a urinary tract infection or pelvic inflammatory disease or ovarian conditions in women.

Upper left abdomen. It's uncommon to experience pain here. When you do, it may suggest a colon, stomach or pancreas problem.

Upper right abdomen. Intense pain in the upper right abdomen is often related to inflammation of the gallbladder (gallbladder attack). The pain may spread to the center of your abdomen and penetrate to your back. Occasionally, an inflamed pancreas or duodenum and sometimes even some liver disorders can produce pain in this area.

Lower left abdomen. Pain here most often suggests a problem in your descending sigmoid colon (just above the rectum). Possible disorders include an infection in the colon (diverticulitis) or inflammation of the colon (Crohn's disease or ulcerative colitis).

Lower right abdomen. Inflammation of the colon also may produce pain in your lower right abdomen. Another possible — and perhaps more serious — cause is appendicitis.

Migrating pain

One of the unusual characteristics of abdominal pain is its ability to travel along deep nerve pathways and emerge at sites away from the source of the problem. Pain related to gallbladder inflammation, for instance, can spread to your chest and along your right shoulder blade, clear up to your right shoulder. Pain from a pancreas disorder may radiate up between your shoulder blades. Your doctor may call this referred pain.

Because of the number of vital organs in your abdomen, and the complex signals they send, it's always a good idea to consult your doctor if you experience the following:

- Severe, recurrent or persistent pain
- Pain that seems to worsen
- Pain accompanied by fever, bleeding or vomiting

It's important to remember that abdominal pain that persists or recurs — regardless of location — can sometimes be due to cancer, especially in older adults.

To learn more

For additional information on conditions that may produce abdominal pain, see these chapters.

- Chapter 6: Ulcers and stomach pain
- Chapter 7: Irritable bowel syndrome
- Chapter 8: Crohn's disease and ulcerative colitis
- Chapter 10: Diverticular disease
- Chapter 11: Gallstones
- Chapter 12: Pancreatitis
- Chapter 13: Liver disease
- Chapter 14: Cancer

Diarrhea and constipation

These are common signs and symptoms that virtually everyone experiences at one time or another. Typically, they last for a short period and then disappear. But sometimes, diarrhea or constipation can be persistent. Persistent signs and symptoms generally mean a digestive disorder.

Diarrhea

Diarrhea is a change toward a more-liquid consistency of your stool, an increased frequency in passing stool, or even an increase in the amount of stool you pass, or often some combination of all three during a given period of time. It may result when the lining of your small intestine becomes inflamed, and your intestines aren't able to absorb nutrients and fluids. Ordinarily after a meal, nutrients and fluids from the food and liquid you've consumed are absorbed in your small intestine. Your colon then absorbs the remaining liquid from digested food particles, forming semisolid stools. Diarrhea occurs when this process is disrupted. It can happen in the following ways.

Viral infection. This is the most common cause of diarrhea. An invading virus can damage the mucous membrane that lines your small intestine, disrupting fluid and nutrient absorption. Typically, after one to three days, symptoms begin to improve and the diarrhea gradually disappears.

Bacterial infection. Bacteria in contaminated food or water can form a toxin that causes your intestinal cells to secrete salt and water. This overwhelms the capacity of your lower small intestine and colon to absorb fluid. As with a viral infection, diarrhea usually lasts one to three days.

Other infectious agents. Though much less common, diarrhea may result from a parasite. Once the parasite is eliminated, the diarrhea usually disappears.

Medications. Diarrhea may also commonly result from medications such as certain antacids that contain magnesium hydroxide. It may also result from taking certain antibiotics. Once the medication is discontinued, the diarrhea usually goes away.

Intestinal disorder. Diarrhea that persists or recurs frequently is usually related to an intestinal disorder. Possible causes include irritable bowel syndrome or an inflammatory disease such as ulcerative colitis or Crohn's disease, or a malabsorption problem such as lactose intolerance or celiac disease. Sometimes diarrhea is associated with a tumor.

Excessive caffeine or alcohol. Caffeine and alcohol can stimulate the passage of stool. If you drink them in excess, they may cause food waste to move through your small intestine and colon too quickly.

Self-care

Diarrhea ordinarily clears up on its own, without the need for antibiotics or other medications. Over-the-counter products, such as Imodium, Pepto-Bismol and Kaopectate, may slow diarrhea, but they won't always speed your recovery. Take these measures to prevent dehydration and reduce symptoms while you recover.

Drink eight to 10 glasses of clear liquids daily. This includes water, weak tea, diluted juices, or beverages containing electrolytes, such as Gatorade or Powerade.

Gradually add solid foods. Begin with easily digestible food such as crackers, toast, rice, cereal and chicken.

Avoid certain foods and beverages. Wait a few days before consuming dairy products, fatty foods, spicy foods, or beverages containing caffeine or alcohol. They can prolong diarrhea.

Don't take antacids containing magnesium. Magnesium can cause diarrhea.

Reduce stress. For some forms of chronic diarrhea, therapies such as acupuncture, acupressure or massage may reduce symptoms by relieving stress and stimulating your body's natural defense systems. However, none of these therapies has been scientifically proved.

Constipation

One of your colon's main jobs is to absorb water from food residue. As food waste stays in your colon, it progressively loses water content. Over time, the waste becomes very dry and difficult to pass.

How long between bowel movements is too long? It varies. Some people have two or three bowel movements each day. Others have bowel movements only three or four times a week. However, if you have bowel movements just once or twice a week, or you have to strain to pass stool, chances are you're constipated.

Constipation can occur for many reasons, and it tends to become more common with age. As you get older, muscles in your digestive tract may become less active. Your lifestyle also may change. Factors that increase your risk of constipation include not drinking enough liquids, eating too little fiber and getting too little exercise.

In addition, certain medications can slow digestion, producing constipation. They include narcotics and antacids containing aluminum. Some people with irritable bowel syndrome experience alternating episodes of diarrhea and constipation.

Generally, constipation is a temporary condition that can be easily corrected. However, there are times when constipation may point to a more serious problem. See your doctor if you experience:

- Recent, unexplained onset of constipation
- Recent, unexplained change in bowel patterns or habits
- Constipation that lasts longer than seven days, despite changes in diet or exercise
- Blood in stool or intense abdominal pain

Self-care

These tips often can help relieve or prevent constipation.

Drink eight to 10 glasses of liquid daily. Liquid helps keep your stool soft. Water is preferable.

Eat high-fiber foods. Fiber helps bulk up and soften stool so that it passes smoothly through your digestive tract. If you're a woman age 50 or under, try to eat 25 grams (g) of fiber daily. If you're a woman over 50, try for 21 g a day. For men age 50 and under, the goal is 38 g. For men over 50, it's 30 g. Whole grains, fruits and vegetables are your best fiber sources (see "Where to find fiber" on page 15).

To avoid abdominal gas, cramping and bloating that can occur from adding too much fiber to your diet too quickly, it's best to gradually increase the amount of fiber you eat over a period of several weeks.

Enjoy regular meals. Eating on a regular schedule promotes normal bowel function.

Exercise regularly. Exercise stimulates digestive muscles, hastening the passage of food through your digestive tract. Try to exercise for 30 to 60 minutes most, if not all, days of the week.

Heed nature's call. The longer you delay going to the bathroom once you feel the urge, the more water that's absorbed from stool and the harder it becomes. Don't linger on the toilet, but relax and give yourself enough time to complete your bowel movement.

Reduce stress. Stress can slow digestion. For some forms of

What about over-the-counter products?

Changes in your lifestyle are the best and safest way to manage constipation. If they don't help, or their effects are limited, you might try a natural fiber supplement, such as psyllium (Metamucil) or methycellulose (Citrucel). These products often relieve constipation within one to three days. Fiber supplements are generally safe, but because they're so absorbent, take them with plenty of water. If you don't drink enough water, the supplements can become constipating — the opposite of what you want.

Laxatives also relieve constipation, but talk to your doctor before taking any laxative. If used for more than a few days, laxatives can be harmful. Stool softeners, such as Colace, Correctol, Stool Softener and Surfak, are the most gentle products. Saline laxatives, such as Milk of Magnesia, also are relatively safe. Stimulant laxatives, including Dulcolax, Ex-Lax and Senokot, are the most powerful.

chronic constipation, practices such as yoga, massage, acupressure or aromatherapy may reduce symptoms by relieving stress and promoting relaxation. However, none of these therapies has been scientifically proved.

To learn more
For additional information on conditions that may produce diarrhea or constipation, see these chapters.
- Chapter 7: Irritable bowel syndrome
- Chapter 8: Crohn's disease and ulcerative colitis
- Chapter 9: Celiac disease
- Chapter 10: Diverticular disease
- Chapter 12: Pancreatitis
- Chapter 14: Cancer

Bleeding

Bleeding from either end of your digestive tract can be alarming. Sometimes the bleeding may be a minor problem, such as gum disease or hemorrhoids. At other times, bleeding is a warning of a more serious condition, such as an ulcer or cancer. The safest course of action is to see your doctor as soon as possible.

Blood in vomit or saliva

Digestive conditions that may produce blood in vomit or saliva include the following:

- Peptic ulcer
- Tear in the lining of your esophagus
- Inflamed tissue in your esophagus, stomach or small intestine
- Cancer of the esophagus or stomach

The blood is usually bright red. Occasionally, it may appear black or dark brown and resemble coffee grounds, which indicates it has been partly digested in either your stomach or your duodenum. This often indicates a serious problem.

Rectal bleeding

An anal tear (fissure) and hemorrhoids are the most frequent causes of rectal bleeding (see "Harmless but troublesome hemorrhoids" on page 47). The blood usually shows up on toilet tissue or in the toilet bowl water and is bright red.

Other causes of rectal bleeding include inflammation of the colon caused by ulcerative colitis or Crohn's disease. Rectal bleeding can also be a warning of noncancerous growths (polyps) or cancer in the colon. Sometimes, this blood is darker in color and mixed in with stool, producing black, maroon or mahogany-colored stools. Black stools may indicate bleeding from the upper intestine.

To learn more

For additional information on conditions that may produce bleeding, see these chapters.

- Chapter 6: Ulcers and stomach pain
- Chapter 8: Crohn's disease and ulcerative colitis
- Chapter 14: Cancer

Harmless but troublesome hemorrhoids

You may not even know they're there. In other cases, the bleeding, itching or burning pain let you know all too well that you have hemorrhoids.

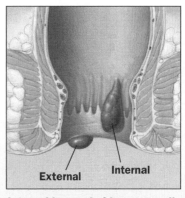

External   Internal

Internal hemorrhoids are usually painless but tend to bleed. External hemorrhoids may cause pain.

Hemorrhoids are blood-engorged veins in your lower rectum. The engorgement results from pressure put on the veins, causing them to form tiny sacs. Hemorrhoids are common. About half of adults have them by age 50.

Constipation and diarrhea are common causes of hemorrhoids. Frequent straining to pass small, hard stools increases pressure on the veins. So does the abrupt expulsion of loose stools. Other causes include lifting heavy objects, obesity, pregnancy, or sitting or standing for long periods.

You can treat most hemorrhoids by increasing fiber and water in your diet, to soften your stools. Soaking in a warm bath for 10 to 15 minutes at least two to three times a day may relieve the swelling and pain. Over-the-counter hemorrhoid creams, ointments or pads containing the astringent witch hazel, or a topical anesthetic agent also can relieve swelling and pain.

Avoid dry, rough toilet paper because it can irritate hemorrhoids. After a bowel movement, clean your anus carefully with a warm washcloth or a medicated wipe.

For troublesome hemorrhoids that won't go away, your doctor may recommend one of the following treatments.

Rubber band ligation. A rubber band is placed around the base of the hemorrhoid inside the rectum. The band cuts off circulation and the hemorrhoid withers away.

Sclerotherapy. A chemical solution is injected around the blood vessel to shrink the hemorrhoid.

Laser coagulation or infrared photocoagulation. These procedures use electrical or laser heat or infrared light to burn and destroy hemorrhoidal tissue.

Hemorrhoidectomy. Surgery is the most effective method for removal of extensive or severe hemorrhoids.

Weight loss

Everyone's weight tends to fluctuate from day to day. But an unintentional loss of more than 5 percent of your weight within one month — or more than 10 percent within six to 12 months — is uncommon. If you're losing weight and you're not sure why, see your doctor.

The possible causes of unexplained weight loss are many. Some digestive conditions that may lead to weight loss include:

- Difficulty swallowing
- Malabsorption disorders
- Pancreas or liver disease
- Cancer

Management of unintentional weight loss first involves determining what's producing the weight loss. Once the cause is known, your doctor is better able to treat the problem. Part of the treatment may involve a high-calorie diet to prevent further weight loss and help you regain weight you've lost.

To learn more

For additional information on conditions that may produce weight loss, see these chapters.

- Chapter 8: Crohn's disease and ulcerative colitis
- Chapter 9: Celiac disease
- Chapter 12: Pancreatitis
- Chapter 13: Liver disease
- Chapter 14: Cancer

Chapter 4

Diagnostic tests

For most people, an occasional bout of heartburn or diarrhea doesn't cause much alarm. It's when digestive symptoms persist or worsen that people usually turn to their doctors. Your doctor may be able to diagnose what's wrong in just a short time. A physical examination, together with questions about your symptoms, eating and exercise habits and daily routine, may be all that's necessary.

Many times, though, before a doctor can make a diagnosis, some tests are needed. Diagnostic tests are especially helpful when your symptoms point to any number of possible causes. These tests can also help confirm your doctor's initial diagnosis.

The type of tests you may undergo will depend on your symptoms and their location, severity and frequency. Here are some of the more common tests for diagnosing digestive problems.

Blood tests

Blood tests often are a first step because they're relatively simple to perform and they give your doctor a general idea of what's going on inside your body. You may have several tests, including one or more of the following.

Complete blood count (CBC). This test measures a number of blood properties, including the amount of red and white cells. A reduction in the number of red blood cells (anemia), and in the hemoglobin found within red blood cells, may be associated with gastrointestinal bleeding. An elevation in white blood cells may indicate an infection or inflammation.

Liver tests. These tests measure certain enzymes and proteins in your blood. If your liver is inflamed or not functioning properly, their levels often are abnormal. For more on tests for liver disease, see Chapter 13.

Carotene, B-12 and folate measurements. Abnormal levels of these nutrients in your blood suggest that your intestines may not be absorbing the nutrients from food (malabsorption problem).

Electrolyte measurements. Severe vomiting or diarrhea can cause an abnormality in the levels of the electrolytes sodium and potassium in your blood. A very low level of potassium can put you at risk of heart problems.

Urine and stool tests

A urine test can sometimes help pinpoint rare causes of abdominal pain or diarrhea by identifying abnormal levels of specific substances excreted in your urine.

If you have severe diarrhea, your doctor may request a stool sample to check for parasites or bacteria (or their associated toxins) that may be causing the diarrhea. Stool tests can also identify increased levels of fat in stool, suggesting a malabsorption problem.

Another common stool test is a fecal occult blood test (Hemoccult test). It checks for hidden (occult) blood that may be linked to cancer or other diseases that can cause intestinal bleeding, such as ulcers or inflammatory bowel disease.

A fecal occult blood test may be a routine part of colorectal cancer screening for people age 50 or older. However, not all cancers bleed, and those that do often bleed intermittently. Therefore, you can get a negative test result even though cancer is present. Certain foods also contain chemicals that can produce a false reading. Broccoli, cauliflower and undercooked red meat can cause a false reading, indicating blood in stool when there isn't any. Just the opposite, vitamin C supplements can mask a positive reaction.

A similar test for blood in stool, called the HemoQuant test, was developed at Mayo Clinic. It's less likely to give false readings. However, it's more expensive, and administering the test is more involved.

Many doctors, including physicians at Mayo Clinic, recommend other screening methods for colorectal cancer instead of, or in addition to, a fecal occult blood test. They include colonoscopy or sigmoidoscopy combined with a colon X-ray.

DNA stool test

A promising new screening test for colorectal cancer is being studied that involves examining stool samples for evidence of DNA markers such as mutated genes. Mutations in several genes have been linked to colorectal cancer. Researchers at Mayo Clinic and other institutions have found that cellular DNA which contains these markers is detectable in stool samples from people with colorectal tumors. In clinical trials to date, stool DNA screening has been effective in detecting the presence of both precancerous polyps (adenomas) and early colorectal cancer (carcinoma). The test requires no bowel preparation, special diet or medication, and just one stool specimen is required per screening. It's hoped that such noninvasive testing will prompt more people to seek screening for colorectal cancer.

X-rays

These tests are another first step in diagnosing digestive problems because like blood tests, they're also relatively simple to perform. The type of X-ray you receive will depend on the location of your symptoms.

Upper gastrointestinal X-ray
This test uses X-ray images to look for problems in your esophagus, stomach and the first part of the small intestine (duodenum). Fasting before the procedure helps clear food and eliminate liquid

from your stomach. This makes it easier to see abnormalities.

A radiologist will position an X-ray machine above you, if you're lying down, or in front of you, if you're standing. At the beginning of the procedure, you swallow a thick, white liquid containing barium. Barium is a soft, metallic alkaline chemical that temporarily coats the lining of your digestive tract and makes the lining show up more clearly on X-ray films. You may also be asked to swallow gas-producing liquid or pills, such as sodium bicarbonate. This stretches the stomach, separating its folds and providing a better view of the inner lining.

The radiologist follows the progress of the barium through your stomach on a video monitor. Watching the flow of barium allows the radiologist to detect problems in how your digestive system works. For instance, X-rays can show if the muscles that control swallowing are functioning properly as they contract and relax. X-ray images also can detect a tumor, an ulcer, or a narrowing (stricture) of your esophagus.

The upper gastrointestinal (GI) X-ray procedure itself may take 20 to 45 minutes, depending on what the radiologist sees. The barium eventually passes through your entire digestive system, producing white stools for a few days. Constipation is sometimes a side effect, which may be prevented by drinking plenty of fluids for a few days afterward. Your doctor may recommend that you use laxatives, enemas or a combination of the two to help eliminate the barium.

Small intestine (small bowel) X-ray
If your doctor suspects that you may have a problem in your small intestine, such as an obstruction, an upper GI X-ray may be expanded to include your entire small intestine. X-ray images are generally taken at 15- to 30-minute intervals as the barium moves through your intestine. It can take up to four hours from the time you drink the barium until it reaches the last portion of the small intestine (terminal ileum). Once the barium reaches your colon, the test is finished. You may be told to use a laxative or enemas to help clear the barium.

Colon X-ray (barium enema)

This test allows your doctor to examine your entire colon with X-rays, to look for ulcers, narrowed areas (strictures), growths of the lining (polyps), small pouches in the lining (diverticula), cancer and other abnormalities.

A colon X-ray is another name for a barium enema. Barium is delivered into your colon through a tube inserted in your rectum. Your colon needs to be empty for this procedure, so for one to two days beforehand you may need to restrict your diet to clear liquids, such as broth, gelatin, coffee, tea and soft drinks. You may also be given laxatives, and perhaps enemas, before the test to help empty your colon.

During a colon X-ray you lie down on your side beneath an X-ray machine. The radiologist places a lubricated, slender tube into your rectum. This tube is connected to a bag of barium that coats the walls of your colon so that its lining will show up more clearly on X-ray. As the barium slowly drains into your colon from the bag above you, you'll feel the urge to have a bowel movement. A small balloon attached to the tube, located in your lower colon or rectum, helps keep the barium from coming back out.

The radiologist will see your colon's shape and condition on a television monitor attached to the X-ray machine. As barium fills your colon, you will be asked to turn and hold several positions to provide different views of your colon. At times, the radiologist may manipulate your colon by pressing firmly on your abdomen and lower pelvis. The radiologist also may inject air through the tubing to expand your colon and improve the image. This is called a double- or air-contrast barium enema.

After the exam, which generally takes about 30 to 45 minutes, the radiologist will lower the barium bag, allowing much of the barium to drain out of your colon. This will make you feel more comfortable. For a few days afterward, you'll probably have white or gray stools while the rest of the barium leaves your system. Drink plenty of liquids during this time to prevent constipation. Your doctor may suggest that you use enemas or take a laxative to help clear out the barium.

Computerized tomography

Computerized tomography (CT) is an effective means of diagnosing tumors, collections of blood or other fluids, or infections (abscesses) deep inside your body. It combines X-rays with computer technology to produce clear, three-dimensional pictures of your internal organs, bone and other tissues.

You lie on an examination table that slides into a doughnut-shaped X-ray scanner. The scanner rotates around you, taking a series of very thin X-rays from many angles. The computer formulates the pictures together into an image that the radiologist can examine from any angle, or can dissect and view layer by layer. CT scans of your abdomen and pelvis can help identify abnormalities in your pancreas, liver, kidneys and, sometimes, your intestines, gallbladder and bile ducts.

An abdominal CT scan is painless. The most uncomfortable part is drinking, or receiving by injection, a liquid containing iodine that makes your organs and tissues show up more clearly. Because some people are allergic to iodine, before the test begins you'll be asked if you've ever had an allergic reaction to iodine. You may also need to fast before having a CT scan. This makes it easier to see the organs and abnormalities.

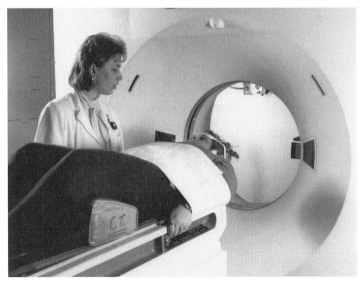

During a computerized tomography (CT) scan, an X-ray scanner rotates around you, taking images of a certain area of your body from various angles.

Ultrasound

Ultrasound procedures combine high-frequency sound waves and computer technology to provide pictures of your internal organs. While you lie on an examining table, a wand-like device (transducer) is placed on your abdomen. The transducer sends out inaudible sound waves that are reflected like sonar. A computer translates those reflected sound waves into a moving, two-dimensional image. The exam is painless and usually takes less than 30 minutes.

Ultrasound is often used to examine abdominal organs such as your liver, pancreas, gallbladder and kidneys. It's especially useful in detecting gallstones and showing the shape, texture and makeup of tumors and cysts. Using special techniques, ultrasound also can determine the flow of blood in arteries and veins, helping to identify a blockage.

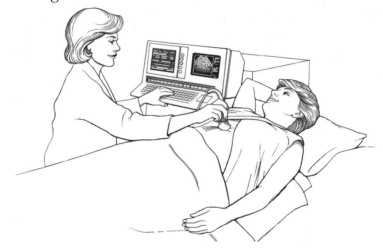

An ultrasound technologist (sonographer) places a hand-held instrument called a transducer against your skin and slowly passes it over the area of your body being examined.

Endoscopy

One of the most effective ways to diagnose digestive problems is to look inside the digestive tract. To do this, a thin, flexible tube with a fiber-optic light and a tiny electronic camera is inserted in one of two ways — either through your mouth and then down through your esophagus, stomach and upper small intestine, or up through your anus and threaded through your rectum and all or a portion of your colon. An endoscope (EN-do-skope) is the instrument that examines the gastrointestinal tract. When used to examine the lower gastrointestinal tract, it's typically referred to as a colonoscope (ko-LON-o-skope) or sigmoidoscope (sig-MOI-do-skope). A sigmoidoscope is shorter than a colonoscope.

Upper endoscopy

This procedure (esophagogastroduodenoscopy, or EGD) lets your doctor look directly inside your esophagus, stomach and duodenum. It can help determine what might be causing signs and symptoms such as difficulty swallowing, heartburn, nausea, vomiting, chest pain, bleeding or upper abdominal pain. Small instruments may also be inserted through the endoscope to perform additional procedures.

During upper endoscopy your doctor may do one or more of the following:
- Look for inflamed tissue, ulcers and abnormal growths
- Take tissue samples (biopsies)
- Remove foreign objects or noncancerous growths (polyps)
- Stretch (dilate) your esophagus if it's narrowed by scar tissue
- Identify and treat bleeding lesions

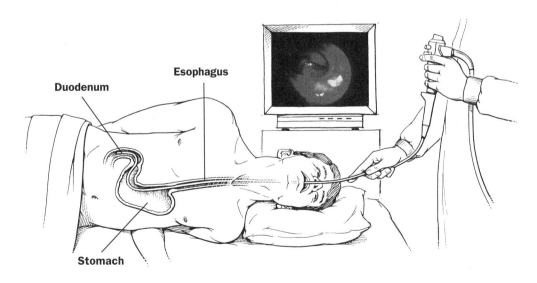

An endoscope provides a real-time image of your upper gastrointestinal tract, including your esophagus, stomach and duodenum. Images from inside the tract appear on a television monitor.

Your stomach needs to be empty for the test, so you can't eat or drink anything for at least four to six hours before the examination. Right before the procedure, you may receive an anesthetic spray to numb your throat and help prevent you from gagging. Most people also receive medication through a vein to sedate them.

After placing the endoscope in your mouth, your doctor will ask you to swallow to help pass the tube from your throat into your esophagus. The tube doesn't interfere with your breathing, but you feel of mild pressure or fullness as it moves down your digestive tract. The small camera transmits a picture, allowing your doctor to carefully examine the lining of your upper digestive tract. Your doctor often can see abnormalities that don't show up as well on an X-ray image, such as inflamed or damaged esophageal tissue from reflux of stomach acid, or small ulcers or tumors in your stomach or duodenum. The device can blow air into your stomach to inflate it, stretching out its natural folds and providing a better view of your stomach lining. The air may cause you to belch or pass gas later.

Upper endoscopy usually takes about 30 minutes, but you generally need an hour or so to recover from the sedative. You'll also need someone to drive you home, since the effects of the sedative may linger for several hours. The endoscope can sometimes cause the throat to feel mildly sore or irritated for a day or two.

Colonoscopy

Similar to the manner in which upper endoscopy is performed, colonoscopy lets your doctor view the inside of your colon. During the exam, your doctor can:

- Inspect the colon for abnormalities, such as bleeding, inflammation, tumors, pouches (diverticula) or narrowed areas
- Take biopsy samples
- Remove polyps
- Treat bleeding sites
- Stretch (dilate) narrowed areas

Your colon needs to be empty for this exam. So, just as with a colon X-ray, you'll be placed on a clear-liquid diet for one to two days beforehand. You may also be given laxatives, and perhaps an enema.

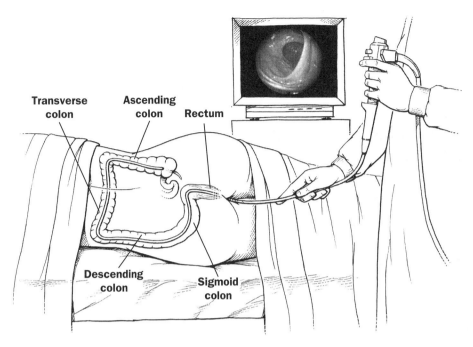

Transverse colon

Ascending colon

Rectum

Descending colon

Sigmoid colon

During colonoscopy a thin, flexible tube is inserted into your rectum and threaded through your colon (large intestine). Images from inside the lower gastrointestinal tract appear on a television monitor.

Before the exam begins, you'll likely receive a sedative through a vein to help you relax. You may also be given a pain reliever. During the exam, you lie on your left side. The colonoscope has a channel that allows your doctor to pump air into your colon. This inflates the colon for a better view of the interior walls.

Colonoscopy on average takes about 30 minutes, but may take longer depending on whether additional procedures — such as polyp removal — are done. You'll feel some abdominal cramping or pressure during the exam, which should end when the scope is removed. Once the exam is over, it takes about an hour to recover from the sedative. You'll also need someone to drive you home because it can take up to a day for the full effects of the sedative to wear off. You may have some bloating and gas for a few hours afterward until you expel the injected air.

Sigmoidoscopy

In this procedure, your doctor examines just your rectum and sigmoid colon, and perhaps part of the descending colon, rather than the entire colon. Sigmoidoscopy is performed in the same manner as

Virtual colonoscopy

Computerized tomography (CT) colonography is a new technique for examining the colon. Sometimes referred to as virtual colonoscopy, it provides two- and three-dimensional images of your colon and rectum without having to use a colonoscope or sedation. Typically, it's used for screening people who are at average risk of colorectal cancer, and for those unable to tolerate a traditional colonoscopy.

Before the scan, you're given laxatives to clear your colon of stool. Your colon is filled with air or carbon dioxide by inserting a small catheter inside the rectum. Images are then made of the entire colon and rectum with a CT scanner. CT colonoscopy is usually faster than traditional colonoscopy. A scan of your entire colon generally takes about 10 minutes. At times you may be asked to hold your breath to limit your abdominal movement and avoid distorting the images. In some cases, a contrast dye is given intravenously to highlight polyps in the colon.

A recent study comparing results of CT colonoscopy with traditional colonoscopy found that the new procedure identified more than 90 percent of polyps 0.3 inches in diameter or larger. However, if suspect areas are found, you'll still need traditional colonoscopy to get a better view of the area, perform biopsies or remove polyps. Researchers are studying whether virtual colonoscopy can be done successfully without prior bowel preparation.

colonoscopy, except that you generally aren't sedated and the only preparation is typically one or two enemas.

Your doctor may order a sigmoid exam to find the cause of diarrhea, abdominal pain, constipation or bleeding, or to look for signs of cancer. Sigmoidoscopy is often a routine part of cancer screening for people at average risk who are age 50 or older. Because growths in the uppermost part of the colon can't be seen with sigmoidoscopy, your doctor may combine the test with a colon X-ray, which shows the entire colon.

Sigmoidoscopy takes only about 10 to 15 minutes, though it can run a few minutes longer if your doctor needs to take any biopsies or treat inflamed or bleeding tissue. You may experience some bloating for a few hours afterward until you expel the injected air. If polyps are found during a sigmoid exam, the next step is generally colonoscopy to remove the polyps and examine the entire colon for additional polyps.

Endoscopic ultrasound

Endoscopic ultrasound (EUS) is a newer form of endoscopic examination that combines endoscopy with ultrasound imaging. EUS creates images of internal organs using ultrasound transmitted from an endoscopic instrument that's positioned within the stomach and bowel. During the EUS examination, an endoscope with both a video camera and an ultrasound probe is passed through your mouth, down your esophagus and into your stomach and sometimes into your small intestine. Ultrasound waves are emitted from the tip of the endoscope, creating reflected images that are projected on a television monitor. This allows your doctor to see through your stomach or intestinal wall and closely examine nearby organs and tissues for disease. EUS also allows your doctor to perform a biopsy of abnormal tissue by passing a fine needle through the stomach or intestinal wall using ultrasound guidance.

This technology is particularly useful in viewing tumors of the esophagus, lungs, stomach, pancreas and rectum, allowing accurate assessment of the size and extent of spread (stage), if malignant. EUS is performed on an outpatient basis and typically takes one to two hours.

Ambulatory acid (pH) probe test

This test can help determine if you have acid reflux, a condition in which stomach acid regurgitates into your esophagus. The test uses an acid-measuring (pH) probe to identify when, and for how long, stomach acid regurgitates into your esophagus.

Insertion of the probe takes about 15 minutes. While you're sitting, a nurse or technician may spray your throat with a numbing medication before the catheter is threaded through your nose (less frequently, your mouth) and into your esophagus. The probe is positioned just above the muscular valve (lower esophageal sphincter) between your esophagus and stomach. A second probe may be placed in your upper esophagus. The catheter doesn't interfere with your breathing, and most people have little or no discomfort.

Connected to the other end of the catheter is a small computer that you wear around your waist or with a strap over your shoulder during the test. It records acid measurements. After the device is in place, you may go home or to the location you're staying. The next day you come back to have the device removed.

Knowing the frequency and duration of acid reflux can help your doctor determine how best to treat the problem. This test also can help determine if reflux may be causing other symptoms, such as chest pain, coughing or wheezing, by correlating episodes of acid reflux with the onset of these symptoms. While wearing the device, you may be asked to record the time you experience signs and symptoms and how long they last.

An ambulatory acid (pH) probe test is sometimes used to determine if treatment to control acid reflux is working. In addition to probes in your upper and lower esophagus, a third probe is placed in your stomach to measure the acid level there.

Esophageal muscle test

This test, called manometry, measures esophageal pressures. It's given if your doctor suspects that you have a swallowing problem caused by muscles in your esophagus that aren't working properly. During manometry (muh-NOM-uh-tre), a tiny, pressure-sensitive tube is inserted through your nose (less frequently, your mouth) and into your esophagus. There, it measures your esophageal muscle contractions as you swallow.

When you swallow, muscles in your esophagus normally contract and relax in rolling waves (peristalsis) that propel food and liquids toward your stomach. In addition, muscular valves at the top and bottom of your esophagus (upper and lower esophageal sphincters) relax and open to let food and liquids pass. They then tighten again to prevent stomach acid from damaging your esophagus and throat. Malfunctions in these muscles can cause difficulty swallowing and lead to gastroesophageal reflux, esophageal spasms, and even pneumonia due to aspiration of stomach contents.

Manometry is most often used after other tests or treatments have failed to identify the problem. The test takes less than an hour. On occasion, manometry may be used to measure pressure in your stomach, small intestine or rectum.

Transit studies

If you have persistent abdominal pain, nausea, vomiting, constipation or diarrhea and other diagnostic tests can't determine a cause, your doctor may order one of several transit studies. These are tests to measure how quickly food passes through certain parts or all of your digestive system. If digestive muscles or nerves aren't working properly, food may move through your system too quickly or too slowly.

Gastric emptying

This test evaluates how quickly your stomach empties food into your small intestine. Your doctor may order this test for unexplained vomiting or if you feel full after eating just a moderate amount of food. For example, if you have diabetes, you could be at risk of gastroparesis (gas-tro-puh-RE-sis), a condition in which your stomach empties too slowly.

After fasting overnight, you visit your doctor and consume some bread, a glass of milk and some eggs. The eggs contain a few drops of a slightly radioactive tracer substance that's clear and tasteless. As you stand or lie on your back, gamma radiation cameras take pictures of the eggs as they pass through your stomach. The pictures don't show your internal organs, only the radioactive eggs. The first pictures are taken right after you eat, followed by pictures at one hour, two hours and four hours. Each session of pictures requires only about five minutes. Between pictures you can sit or walk around.

If your stomach is emptying normally, 11 percent to 39 percent of the eggs will be out of your stomach at one hour, 40 percent to 76 percent at two hours, and 84 percent to 98 percent at four hours.

Gastric emptying and small-bowel transit

This test is the same as the gastric emptying test, except that an additional series of pictures is taken at six hours. If your small intestine is moving the food normally, 46 percent to 98 percent of the eggs will have passed through your small intestine by this time and be in your colon.

Whole-gut transit

This test may be done if your doctor suspects that your digestive tract isn't moving food normally, but he or she is uncertain where the problem is. You begin by swallowing a capsule containing a radioactive tracer element. The capsule is designed to remain intact until it reaches your upper colon, where it dissolves and releases the tracer element that eventually passes through your lower digestive tract.

About an hour after taking the capsule, you eat the same kind of egg breakfast used in other transit studies, followed by the same schedule of pictures as in gastric emptying and small-bowel transit studies. One important difference is that you come back the next day for a picture 24 hours after taking the capsule. By the next morning, the capsule should have released its tracer element, which should be seen mixed in with food residue in the middle or lower colon. If the tracer element remains at the beginning of your colon, your colon isn't propelling food waste normally.

Colonic transit

Your doctor may order this study of only your colon if you have severe, persistent constipation. You take the same kind of capsule given in the whole-gut transit study, but you don't need to eat the specially prepared breakfast. Instead, a nurse or medical technician will tell you when to eat your meals throughout the day. A picture is taken as soon as you swallow the capsule, then four hours later. By the time of the four-hour picture, the capsule should be in the beginning of your colon. You will need to return the next day for a

24-hour picture to see how far the tracer element has progressed. As in the whole-gut study, if the element hasn't made it to your middle or lower colon, your colon isn't moving food fast enough. This would explain your constipation.

Chapter 5

Gastroesophageal reflux disease (GERD)

Nearly everyone has experienced heartburn, that burning sensation in your chest, and sometimes throat, from stomach acid that washes back into your esophagus. It may be because you ate too much at dinner. Or perhaps you didn't let your bedtime snack digest before you hit the pillow.

Key signs and symptoms

- Heartburn
- Acid reflux
- Difficulty swallowing
- Chest pain
- Persistent coughing
- Hoarseness

Heartburn is common, and an occasional episode is generally nothing to worry about. Many people, however, battle heartburn regularly, even daily. About 7 percent of Americans have heartburn every day, and about 10 percent have it weekly. Frequent heartburn can be a serious problem, and it deserves medical attention. Most often, frequent or constant heartburn is a symptom of gastro-esophageal reflux disease (GERD).

What's GERD?

When you eat, food travels down your esophagus to a muscular valve that separates your lower esophagus and stomach. Called the lower esophageal sphincter (LES), this valve opens to allow food to pass into your stomach and then closes again.

Reflux of stomach acid results when the valve weakens and doesn't close as tightly as it should. Stomach acid washes back into your lower esophagus, causing frequent heartburn and disrupting daily life. The acid also may regurgitate to your upper esophagus, leaving a sour taste in your mouth or causing you to cough. This constant backwash of acid can irritate the lining of the esophagus, causing it to inflame (esophagitis). Over time, the inflammation can erode the esophagus, producing bleeding, or narrow the esophagus, causing difficulty swallowing or even breathing problems.

Gastroesophageal reflux disease is the name for chronic acid reflux that causes esophagitis. Anyone can have GERD, even children and infants. Studies show that GERD is no more common in older people than in younger adults. However, its signs and symptoms and their frequency may be more severe in older adults.

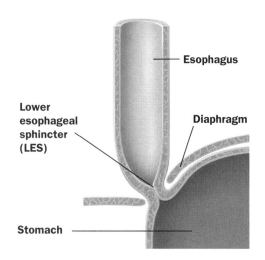

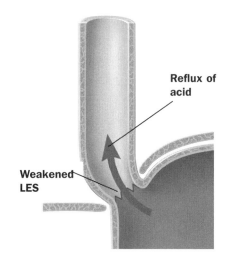

Normally, the lower esophageal sphincter (LES) remains closed, preventing stomach acid from washing up into the esophagus. If the LES becomes weakened or relaxed, acid can enter the esophagus, causing heartburn and tissue inflammation.

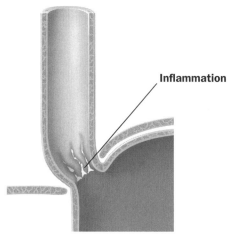

Variation in signs and symptoms

Acid reflux and heartburn are two symptoms that most people with GERD share. But beyond these two, signs and symptoms usually vary and may include the following.

Chest pain. The pain is often worse after a heavy meal or at night. Because GERD and heart disease can coexist, it's important to have chest pain evaluated to make sure it isn't associated with a heart condition.

Coughing. Some people experience a chronic cough, which may be due to small amounts of stomach acid regurgitating into lung airways (bronchi).

Wheezing. Acid reflux appears to worsen, and perhaps even cause wheezing that can resemble asthma.

Throat problems. Acid reflux and inflammation may produce hoarseness, a need to keep clearing your throat, a feeling of a lump in your throat (globus sensation), a chronic sore throat or hiccups.

Difficulty swallowing. Swallowing problems may indicate a narrowing (stricture) of the esophagus or a temporary spasm of the esophagus. In severe cases, you may choke or feel as if food is lodged behind your breastbone.

Bleeding. Inflammation and erosion of the lining of the esophagus or an esophageal ulcer can cause bleeding. The blood may be bright red or darker in color (even black) and appear in vomit or mixed in with stool.

Other causes of esophagitis

The most common cause of an inflamed esophagus (esophagitis) is GERD, but esophagitis can also develop for other reasons. A fungus or a virus can inflame esophageal tissue, especially in people with weakened immune systems. Certain pills also may irritate tissues during swallowing, especially if taken without adequate liquid or while lying down. These include the antibiotics erthromycin and tetracycline, alendronate (Fosamax) taken for osteoporosis, vitamin C tablets, iron and potassium.

Who gets GERD?

It isn't always easy to pinpoint what causes GERD. Some people with the disease don't have any common risk factors that point to a possible cause. Many people, though, have at least one. There are several factors that can significantly increase your risk of GERD.

Hiatal hernia. In this condition, part of your stomach protrudes into your lower chest, and your diaphragm — the large muscle that separates your chest and abdomen — is no longer able to support the lower esophageal sphincter (see "What's a hiatal hernia" on page 78). A hiatal hernia can worsen acid reflux.

Certain foods. Caffeine, fats, mint and chewing gum all may contribute to or aggravate GERD.

Being overweight. Many, but not all, people with GERD are overweight. Excess weight puts extra pressure on your stomach and diaphragm, forcing open the lower esophageal sphincter. Eating very large meals or meals high in fat may cause similar effects.

Excessive alcohol. Alcohol reduces pressure on the lower esophageal sphincter, allowing it to relax and open. Alcohol also may irritate the lining of the esophagus.

Smoking. Smoking may increase acid production and aggravate reflux.

Family history. Mayo Clinic researchers believe that a genetic link predisposes some people to the disease. If your parents or siblings have or had GERD, your chances of having the condition are increased.

Other conditions or diseases can aggravate or precipitate symptoms of GERD, although they're generally not considered a cause of GERD.

Pregnancy. GERD is more common during pregnancy because of increased production of progesterone. This hormone relaxes many muscles, including the lower esophageal sphincter. GERD during pregnancy may also occur because of increased pressure on the stomach.

Asthma. GERD is more common in people who have asthma. However, it's unclear if asthma is a cause or an effect of GERD. One theory is that the coughing and sneezing that accompany asthma may lead to pressure changes in your chest and abdomen, causing regurgitation of stomach acid into the esophagus. Some asthma medications used to widen (dilate) airways also may relax the lower esophageal sphincter and allow reflux of acid.

It's also possible that GERD may worsen asthma symptoms. For example, you may inhale (aspirate) small amounts of digestive juices that regurgitate into your esophagus, damaging lung airways.

Diabetes. One of the many complications of diabetes is a disorder in which your stomach takes too long to empty (gastroparesis). Left in your stomach too long, stomach contents can reflux into the esophagus, damaging the lining.

Peptic stomach ulcer. An open sore (ulcer) near the valve that controls the flow of food from your stomach into your small intestine (pylorus, or pyloric valve) can obstruct the valve or keep it from working properly. Food and fluids don't empty from your stomach as fast as they should, causing acid to remain in your stomach longer than normal and back up into your esophagus.

Delayed stomach emptying. In addition to diabetes or an ulcer, abnormal nerve or muscle function can delay emptying of your stomach, causing acid backup.

Connective tissue disorders. Diseases that cause muscular tissue to thicken and swell can keep digestive muscles from relaxing and contracting as they should, allowing acid reflux. Scleroderma is an example.

Zollinger-Ellison syndrome. One of the complications of this rare disorder is that your stomach produces extremely high amounts of acid, increasing the risk of acid reflux and GERD.

Danger of ignoring your signs and symptoms

Complications of GERD are fairly common. Left untreated, acid reflux can lead to one or more of the following conditions.

Esophageal narrowing (stricture)
A stricture occurs in about 10 percent of people with GERD. Damage to cells in the lower esophagus from acid exposure (reflux esophagitis) leads to formation of scar tissue. The scar tissue narrows

the food pathway and can interfere with swallowing, causing chunks of food to get caught in the narrowed area. Treatment for a stricture generally consists of a procedure that stretches and widens narrowed esophageal tissues and an acid-suppressing medication to help prevent re-narrowing.

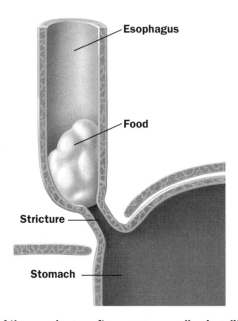

Narrowing (stricture) of the esophagus often causes swallowing difficulties.

Ulcer in the esophagus

Stomach acid can severely erode tissues in the esophagus, causing an open sore to form. The ulcer may bleed, cause pain and make swallowing difficult. Medications and lifestyle changes to control stomach acid reflux can cure an ulcer by giving damaged tissues time to heal. See Chapter 6 for more information on ulcers.

Barrett's esophagus

This is a serious complication of GERD. Although uncommon, Barrett's esophagus is increasing in incidence. In this condition, the color and composition of the tissue lining the lower esophagus change. Instead of pink, it turns a salmon color. Under a microscope, instead of the normal, flat tile-shaped cells, the cells in Barrett's tissue are tall and resemble shag carpet. This cellular change is called metaplasia.

Metaplasia is brought on by repeated and long-term exposure to stomach acid and is associated with an increased risk of esophageal cancer. Between 5 percent and 15 percent of people with GERD have Barrett's esophagus. Once you have it, your chance of having esophageal cancer are 30 to 125 times as high as that of the general population. However, because esophageal cancer is uncommon, the risk of someone with GERD getting cancer is very low.

Endoscopy is the most common procedure for identifying Barrett's esophagus. A thin, flexible tube that contains a tiny camera is inserted down your throat, allowing your doctor to examine your esophagus for tissue damage. Your doctor may remove small pieces of tissue (biopsy) from your lower esophagus and have them examined for evidence of precancerous cellular changes (dysplasia). The degree of precancerous changes in Barrett's esophagus ranges from none, to small but noticeable changes (low-grade dysplasia), to

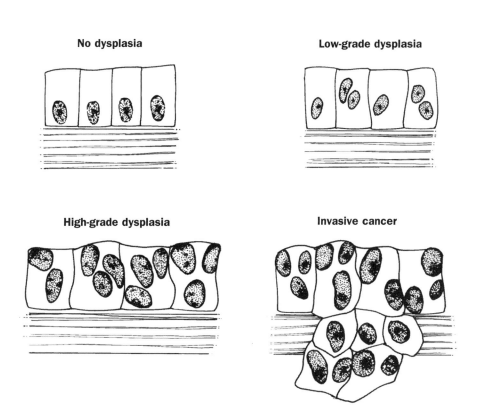

With Barrett's esophagus, cells lining the esophagus can change in size, shape and organization. The more noticeable the changes, the greater the risk of cancer developing in the cells and invading other structures.

serious changes (high-grade dysplasia), and finally, to invasive cancer. The more serious the changes, the greater the risk that cancer is present or will develop.

Treatment is available for Barrett's esophagus. The problem is that people often see a doctor too late, after cancer is already present. Treatment begins by controlling GERD through diet and lifestyle changes and, often, taking medications to control reflux of stomach acid. Your doctor may also recommend an endoscopic examination every two to three years to monitor changes in esophageal tissues. If you have high-grade dysplasia, treatment may involve surgery to remove a portion of your esophagus. Another option may involve the burning away of damaged tissue.

See your doctor

If you experience heartburn at least twice a week for several weeks, or your symptoms seem to be getting worse, see your doctor. He or she will ask about your health and your symptoms. How often do they occur? When do they usually occur? Have they become more severe? Are there things that seem to make them better? Your doctor may also ask about your lifestyle. Do you smoke? What are your eating habits? Have you gained weight recently? How much alcohol do you drink?

If you have the typical symptoms of GERD — heartburn and acid reflux — and you don't have any other symptoms or complications, you may not need any tests. However, if your heartburn is severe or you have additional signs and symptoms including unexplained weight loss or difficulty swallowing (dysphagia), you may be experiencing complications. You'll probably need some tests before your doctor can make a diagnosis.

To diagnose GERD and identify complications, your doctor may recommend one or more of the following tests.

Upper endoscopy. It's the most accurate because it allows your doctor to see your esophagus and stomach. Your doctor can also take biopsies, if necessary.

Upper gastrointestinal X-ray. It can detect abnormalities or obstruction in your upper gastrointestinal tract. Before this test, you drink a white solution (barium) that coats your digestive tract, making your esophagus and stomach more visible on X-ray films.

Ambulatory acid (pH) probe test. It measures the amount of time during the day and night that stomach acid is present in your upper and lower esophagus. It can also help determine the frequency and duration of acid reflux.

Chapter 4 has details on these tests and how they're performed.

Treatment begins with self-care

Regardless of the severity of your disease, the first step in managing GERD is to examine your lifestyle. For mild symptoms, a change in habits might be at least part of what's needed to manage the disease. For more severe symptoms, lifestyle changes may make your condition easier to control along with medication.

Quit smoking. Smoking increases acid reflux and can dry up saliva. Saliva helps to protect your esophagus from stomach acid.

Eat smaller meals. This reduces pressure on the lower esophageal sphincter, helping to prevent the valve from opening and acid from washing back into your esophagus.

Sit up after you eat. Wait at least three hours before going to bed or taking a nap. By then, most of the food in your stomach will have emptied into the small intestine so that it can't flow back into your esophagus.

Don't exercise immediately after a meal. Wait two to three hours before engaging in strenuous physical activity.

Limit fatty foods. Studies show a potentially strong link between consumption of fat and GERD. Fatty foods relax the lower esophageal sphincter, allowing stomach acid into the esophagus. Fat also slows stomach emptying, increasing the length of time acid can regurgitate.

Avoid problem foods and beverages. These may include caffeinated drinks, chocolate, onions, spicy foods and mint. They tend to increase production of stomach acid and may relax the lower esophageal sphincter. Also limit citrus fruits and tomato-based foods. They're acidic and can irritate an inflamed esophagus, making GERD symptoms worse in some people.

If your lower esophageal sphincter is moderately to severely weakened, it doesn't matter what you eat or drink. Stomach acid backs up into the esophagus regardless of what's in your stomach.

Limit or avoid alcohol. Alcohol relaxes the lower esophageal sphincter and may irritate the esophagus, worsening symptoms.

Lose excess weight. Heartburn and acid regurgitation are more likely to occur when there's added pressure on your stomach from excess weight.

Raise the head of your bed 6 to 9 inches. This provides a gradual incline from your feet to your head and helps prevent acid from flowing back into your esophagus as you sleep. Place a foam wedge under the mattress to raise it, or better yet, put blocks of wood under the legs at the head of your bed.

Avoid tightfitting clothes. They put pressure on your stomach.

Take time to relax. When you're under stress, digestion slows, worsening GERD symptoms. Although not scientifically proved, relaxation techniques, such as deep breathing, meditation or yoga, may improve GERD by reducing stress.

Drugs and supplements that can worsen GERD

Some medications and supplements can aggravate symptoms of GERD by reducing lower esophageal sphincter pressure or irritating the esophagus. If possible, try to avoid the following medications or supplements. If you're already taking one or more of these, talk with your doctor first before you quit taking it. Suddenly stopping its use could be dangerous to your health.

- Anticholinergics, medications that relax smooth muscle
- Calcium channel blockers, medications for high blood pressure
- Potassium tablets
- Vitamin C tablets
- Tetracycline, an antibiotic in capsule form
- Nonsteroidal anti-inflammatory drugs, such as aspirin, ibuprofen (Advil, Motrin, others) naproxen (Aleve) and ketoprofen (Orudis)
- Quinidine (Quinidex), a heart-arrhythmia medication
- Sedatives and tranquilizers
- Alendronate (Fosamax), an osteoporosis medication

Medications that can help

Perhaps you've tried everything. You've cut back on fatty foods, you're eating smaller meals, you've lost some weight, and you don't smoke. Yet your symptoms continue or have improved only slightly. When lifestyle changes aren't effective, the next step may be medication.

Antacids
These over-the-counter medications are best suited for occasional or mild heartburn. Antacids neutralize gastric acid and can provide quick, temporary relief. They come in a variety of forms with neutralizing agents. For example, Tums and Rolaids are chewable tablets that contain calcium carbonate. Mylanta, Maalox and Rolaids contain magnesium or calcium and come in liquid or tablet form. Liquids generally work faster than tablets, but some people find them less convenient.

Antacids can relieve your symptoms, but they won't cure the cause of your reflux. The products are generally safe, but if taken constantly they can cause side effects, such as diarrhea or constipation. Some antacids can also interact with other medications, including medications for kidney or heart disease. Constant use of products containing magnesium may cause a magnesium buildup, which can aggravate or result in kidney disease, especially if you have diabetes. Too much calcium also can result in kidney stones. If you take an antacid regularly, mention this to your doctor.

Acid blockers
Also known as histamine (H-2) blockers, these popular medications are available over the counter and by prescription. Instead of neutralizing acid, they reduce acid secretion. Acid blockers differ from antacids in that they can prevent acid reflux and heartburn, not just relieve it. They're also longer acting, relieving heartburn for up to eight hours, rather than four hours or less for antacids.

Acid blockers include the medications cimetidine (Tagamet), famotidine (Pepcid), nizatidine (Axid) and ranitidine (Zantac).

Over-the-counter acid blockers are half the strength of their prescription counterparts. It's best to take acid blockers before a meal that may give you heartburn. You can also take them after symptoms occur, but it takes about 30 minutes for them to work.

Acid blockers help heal esophagitis and ulcers by reducing exposure of esophageal tissues to acid. Your doctor may recommend that you take an acid blocker for a few months, or longer, if it helps to keep your symptoms at bay. The drugs infrequently cause some side effects, including bowel changes, dry mouth, dizziness or drowsiness, but they're generally safe. However, some acid blockers shouldn't be taken with other medications because of risk of a dangerous interaction. If you take an acid blocker and also use other medications, check with your doctor or pharmacist about possible drug interactions.

Proton pump inhibitors (PPIs)

These medications are the most effective for treatment of GERD. Esomeprazole (Nexium), lansoprazole (Prevacid) and rabeprazole (Aciphex) are available by prescription. Omeprazole (Prilosec) is available over the counter. One proton pump inhibitor, pantoprazole (Protonix), may be taken orally or given intravenously.

PPIs block acid production and allow time for damaged esophageal tissue to heal. PPIs are convenient to use because you generally take them only once a day. However, the drugs are more expensive than other GERD medications.

PPIs are generally safe and well tolerated for long-term treatment of GERD. In trials, PPIs have been found safe to use for at least 10 years. Initial concerns that the medications may lead to serious stomach tumors have not been substantiated. If your GERD is severe, your doctor may recommend the drugs for indefinite use to keep your symptoms under control.

Side effects occur in a small number of people who take PPIs. These side effects may include stomach or abdominal pain, diarrhea, loose stools, headache or lightheadedness during the first few weeks of taking the medication. If the side effects are mild, your dosage may not require an immediate adjustment or discontinuation. People find that side effects usually subside after about three weeks. The drugs may be used in combination with H-2 blockers in people who experience reflux symptoms at night.

Motility (prokinetic) agents

Instead of reducing acid production, these medications increase gastric emptying and increase lower esophageal sphincter pressure. Cisapride (Propulsid) was the most commonly used motility agent. It has been withdrawn from the U.S. market because it posed a greater risk of side effects and adverse drug interactions than other GERD medications. Cisapride may also worsen or cause heart rhythm problems (cardiac arrhythmia).

Another motility agent, metoclopramide (Reglan), works similarly. However, neurologic and other side effects, such as depression, may limit its use. Researchers are working on safer motility drugs.

When surgery may be needed

Because of the effectiveness of medications, surgery for GERD is uncommon. However, it may be an option if you can't tolerate the medications, if the medications are ineffective, or if you can't afford their long-term use. Your doctor may also recommend surgery if you have any of these complications:

- Large hiatal hernia (see "What's a hiatal hernia?" on page 78)
- Severe esophagitis, especially with bleeding
- Recurrent narrowing (stricture) of the esophagus
- Barrett's esophagus, especially with progressive precancerous or cancerous changes
- Severe pulmonary problems, such as bronchitis or pneumonia, due to acid reflux

Before 1991, a procedure called open Nissen fundoplication was the surgery of choice for severe GERD. Today, doctors are able to perform the same surgery with similar success laparoscopically — through a few small abdominal incisions, instead of one large one. The advantages of laparoscopic surgery are a shorter recovery time and less discomfort.

Nissen fundoplication involves tightening the lower esophageal sphincter to prevent reflux by wrapping the very top of the stomach

What's a hiatal hernia?

A hiatal hernia is a protrusion of the upper portion of your stomach into your lower chest cavity. A hiatal hernia was once thought to be the most common cause of gastroesophageal reflux disease, but doctors have taken a different view. Only moderate to large hiatal hernias are thought to play a role in GERD, either by contributing to severe reflux or aggravating GERD symptoms.

Your chest cavity and abdomen are separated by a large, dome-shaped muscle called the diaphragm. A hiatal hernia occurs when the upper stomach pushes upward through the opening (hiatus) in the diaphragm through which the esophagus passes.

A small hiatal hernia isn't likely to cause you problems. In fact, most hiatal hernias cause no symptoms at all. Moderate- or large-sized hernias can contribute to heartburn in one of two ways. Normally, your diaphragm is aligned with your lower esophageal sphincter, supporting and providing pressure on the sphincter to keep it closed. A hiatal hernia displaces the sphincter, reducing pressure on the valve. A hiatal hernia can also cause heartburn if the herniated portion of your stomach becomes a reservoir for gastric acid, which may readily travel up the esophagus.

Pain, bloating, difficulty swallowing or obstruction of your esophagus may occur if the portion of the stomach that protrudes into the chest cavity becomes twisted. In rare cases, a large portion of your stomach may protrude into your chest cavity, restricting blood flow to the stomach. This can produce severe chest pain and difficulty swallowing.

Large hiatal hernias that pose problems are generally treated with surgery to return the stomach to its normal position and close the opening in the diaphragm.

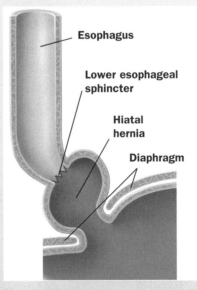

With a hiatal hernia, the top portion of the stomach protrudes above the diaphragm.

Esophagus

Lower esophageal sphincter

Hiatal hernia

Diaphragm

around the outside of the lower esophagus. During laparoscopic surgery, a surgeon makes three to five tiny incisions in the abdomen and inserts small instruments, including a flexible tube with a tiny camera, through the incisions. To provide more space for your surgeon to see and work, your abdomen is inflated with carbon dioxide. The surgery takes about two hours and typically requires a one-or-two day hospital stay.

More than 90 percent of the people who undergo Nissen fundoplication remain free of GERD symptoms for at least one year. In one study, almost 90 percent were symptom-free after five years. These success rates apply to the laparoscopic and open procedures.

Other surgical procedures include Toupet fundoplication, Hill repair and the Belsey Mark IV operation. All involve restructuring the lower esophageal sphincter to improve its strength and ability to prevent reflux. These surgeries are done less often, and their success is often dependent on the skill and experience of the surgeon.

Complications from surgery generally are mild, but may include difficulty swallowing, bloating, diarrhea and a sense of feeling full after eating only a moderate amount (early satiety). These complications generally go away two to three months after surgery.

New, less invasive procedures

The Food and Drug Administration recently approved three procedures for tightening the lower esophageal sphincter that could one day become popular alternatives to long-term use of medication. The new procedures generally take an hour or less to perform, they don't require any incisions, and you can go home the same day. The procedures are performed endoscopically through a long, flexible tube that's inserted into your mouth and threaded down your esophagus.

EndoCinch endoluminal gastroplication. This procedure uses a tool that's like a miniature sewing machine, which is attached to an endoscope. It places pairs of stitches (sutures) in the stomach near the weakened sphincter. The suturing material is tied together, creating barriers (plications) to prevent stomach acid from washing into your esophagus. The barriers are located at and just below the junction of the esophagus and stomach.

Stretta procedure. This approach uses controlled radiofrequency energy to heat and melt (coagulate) tissues deep within the portion of the esophagus that contains the malfunctioning valve and at the junction of the esophagus and upper stomach. The procedure appears to work by creating scar tissue and altering the sensory nerves that respond to refluxed acid.

Studies haven't found any serious side effects from these procedures. However, both may cause a sore throat or chest pain. The long-term effectiveness of the procedures is still unknown.

Neither procedure is recommended if you have a hiatal hernia or Barrett's esophagus. Both procedures are intended for people with uncomplicated GERD who prefer minimally invasive surgery to medications.

Enteryx. This is the simplest of the new, less invasive procedures to treat GERD. Enteryx involves the injection of a compound called ethylene polyvinyl alcohol into the lower esophageal sphincter, just within the stomach. The injection is done with guidance from real-time X-ray. The compound is in liquid form outside the body, but when it comes into contact with tissues inside the body, it turns into an expanding, spongy material. The procedure takes 20 to 30 minutes to perform and some discomfort can be expected. The procedure appears to be as effective as endoluminal gastroplication (EndoCinch) or coagulation of the lower esophageal sphincter (Stretta procedure).

Chapter 6

Ulcers and stomach pain

Too much stress, too much spicy food, and it was thought that you could be headed for an ulcer. Not long ago, the common belief was that ulcers were a result of lifestyle. A great deal has changed. Doctors now know that a bacterial infection or medication, not stress or diet,

Key signs and symptoms

- Gnawing pain in stomach or upper abdomen
- Blood in vomit
- Blood in stool
- Unexplained weight loss
- Pain in the midback

causes most ulcers. And instead of taking months or years to treat, ulcers can often be cured in two to eight weeks.

There's one small catch. Some people who think they have ulcers really don't. Instead, they may have a condition called nonulcer dyspepsia, in which symptoms may mimic those of an ulcer. Unlike ulcers, which are decreasing in number, cases of nonulcer dyspepsia appear to be on the rise.

An open sore

Ulcer is the medical term for an open sore. There are several types of ulcers. One is a pressure ulcer (bedsore, or decubitus ulcer) that can occur on your lower back or buttocks from lying too long in one position. Another is a stasis ulcer that can develop on an ankle from slowing of blood flow. The most common type of ulcer, however — and the type that people generally associate with the term *ulcer* — is a peptic ulcer. Peptic ulcers develop on the inside lining of the stomach or small intestine. About 10 percent of Americans experience a peptic ulcer at some point in their lives.

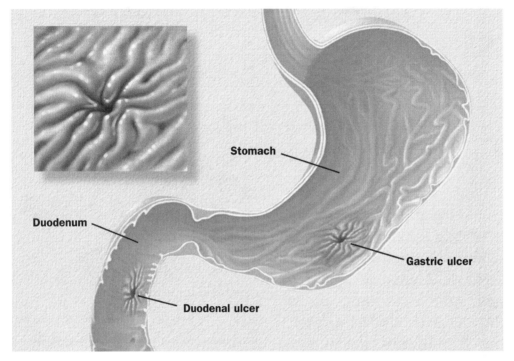

A peptic ulcer is a sore in the lining of your stomach or small intestine. A peptic ulcer located in your stomach is called a gastric ulcer. A peptic ulcer in the small intestine most often occurs in the duodenum and is called a duodenal ulcer.

A peptic ulcer that occurs in your stomach is called a gastric ulcer. If the ulcer develops in your small intestine, it's named for the section of the intestine where it develops. The most common is a duodenal (doo-o-DEE-nul) ulcer, which develops in the duodenum, the first part of the small intestine.

Left untreated, peptic ulcers can cause internal bleeding and can create a hole in the wall of your stomach or small intestine, putting you at risk of serious inflammation or infection of your abdominal cavity (peritonitis). Peptic ulcers can also produce scar tissue that can obstruct passage of food through the digestive tract and cause weight loss.

The most common symptom of a peptic ulcer is a gnawing pain in your upper abdomen between your navel and breastbone (sternum). This pain, caused by stomach acid washing over the open sore, may linger for just a few minutes, or it may last for hours. The pain is often worse when your stomach is empty, and therefore the pain tends to flare at night. Food buffers the acid. That's why eating often temporarily relieves the pain. Because they eat often, some people with ulcers experience weight gain.

Other signs and symptoms include vomiting up blood, which may appear bright red or black like coffee grounds, and dark colored blood mixed with stool. Ulcers also can cause midback pain.

Bacteria a common culprit

A major breakthrough in the understanding and treatment of peptic ulcers occurred in 1983 when two Australian researchers found a corkscrew-shaped bacterial organism in biopsy specimens of people who had ulcers and persistent stomach inflammation (gastritis).

The bacterium discovered by the researchers, called *Helicobacter pylori (H. pylori)*, lives and multiplies within the mucous layer that covers and protects tissues that line the stomach and small intestine. Often, *H. pylori* causes no problems. But sometimes it can erode digestive tissues, producing an ulcer. Approximately one in five people infected with *H. pylori* gets an ulcer. One reason may be that these people already have damage to the lining of their stomachs or small intestines, making it easier for bacteria to invade and infect tissues.

Although it's not clear how the organism spreads, it appears to be transmitted from person to person by close contact. Poor food handling and sanitation practices are thought to be common routes of transmission. Because scientists have found *H. pylori* in water, they suspect the infection may also be transmitted in contaminated drinking water.

Risk factors include:
- Being born in a developing country
- Having a low socioeconomic standard of living
- Living in a large family or crowded conditions

- Having an infant in the home
- Being exposed to vomit of an infected individual

The good news is that the rate of new *H. pylori* infection seems to be dropping in the United States. Children raised in the 1920s to the 1940s are much more likely to have been infected than are today's children. About 50 percent of people older than 60 have *H. pylori*, while only about 20 percent of Americans under age 40 are infected with it.

Major factors that may have contributed to the decrease in *H. pylori* infection are improvements in socioeconomic status and sanitation, and widespread use of antibiotics in children. Treating conditions such as ear infections and other common childhood illnesses with antibiotics may have done double duty by preventing or treating *H. pylori* early in life.

Other causes of ulcers

H. pylori is the most common, but not the only, cause of peptic ulcers. *H. pylori* presently accounts for about two-thirds of all peptic ulcers in the United States. The rate of *H. pylori* infection is higher in areas in which people live in poverty and in crowded conditions than it is in other parts of the country.

Besides *H. pylori*, there are other causes of peptic ulcers.

Regular use of pain relievers

Nonsteroidal anti-inflammatory drugs (NSAIDs) can irritate or inflame the lining of your stomach and small intestine. The medications are available by prescription and over the counter. Non-prescription NSAIDs include aspirin, ibuprofen (Advil, Motrin, others), naproxen (Aleve) and ketoprofen (Orudis). To help avoid digestive upset, take NSAIDs with meals.

Between 15 percent and 30 percent of people who regularly take NSAIDs develop ulcers. The drugs inhibit production of an enzyme (cyclooxygenase) that produces prostaglandins. These hormone-like substances help protect your stomach lining from chemical and physical injury. Without this protection, stomach acid can erode the lining, causing bleeding and ulcers. On the other hand, the pain reliever acetaminophen (Tylenol, others) doesn't inhibit the production of prostaglandins and doesn't cause stomach ulcers.

It's uncertain, but possible, that regular use of NSAIDs may also increase the risk of ulcers in people infected with *H. pylori*.

Smoking

Nicotine in tobacco increases the volume and concentration of stomach acid, increasing your risk of an ulcer. Tobacco use may also slow healing during ulcer treatment.

Excessive alcohol

Alcohol can irritate and erode the mucous lining of your stomach and intestines, causing inflammation and bleeding. It's uncertain, however, whether this alone can progress into an ulcer or whether other contributing factors must be present, such as *H. pylori* bacteria or nicotine.

Diagnosing an ulcer

An ulcer is generally discovered one of two ways. Your doctor may begin with an upper gastrointestinal (GI) X-ray outlining your stomach and duodenum. Before the X-ray, you swallow a white, liquid (barium) that coats your digestive tract and makes an ulcer more visible. An upper GI X-ray can detect some ulcers, but not all.

Endoscopy may follow an upper GI X-ray if the X-ray suggests a possible ulcer, or your doctor may perform endoscopy in place of an X-ray. In this more sensitive procedure, a long, narrow tube with an attached camera is threaded down your throat into your stomach and duodenum. With this instrument, your doctor can view your upper digestive tract and identify an ulcer. If an ulcer is found, your doctor may remove small tissue samples (biopsy) near the ulcer. These samples are examined under a microscope to rule out cancer of the stomach. A biopsy can also identify the presence of *H. pylori* in your stomach lining. Because cancer of the duodenum is rare, a biopsy of a duodenal ulcer is seldom necessary. See Chapter 4 for details on endoscopy and upper GI X-rays.

In addition to a biopsy, three other tests can determine if the cause of your ulcer is *H. pylori* infection.

Blood test. It checks for the presence of *H. pylori* antibodies. A disadvantage of this test is that it can't differentiate between past exposure and current infection. After *H. pylori* bacteria have been eradicated, you may still get a positive result.

Breath test. This test uses a radioactive carbon atom to detect *H. pylori*. First, you blow into a small plastic bag, which is then sealed. Second, you drink a small glass of a clear, tasteless liquid. The liquid contains radioactive carbon as part of a substance (urea) that will be broken down by *H. pylori.* Thirty minutes later, you blow into a second bag which also is then sealed. If you're infected with *H. pylori,* your second breath sample will contain the radioactive carbon in the form of carbon dioxide. It takes about a day to get the test results.

If you're taking a medication called a proton pump inhibitor, you'll need to stop taking the medication for at least three days before the breath test because the medication can interfere with the test results.

The breath test is accurate 96 percent to 98 percent of the time. That's similar to the blood test. The advantage of the breath test is that it can monitor the effectiveness of treatment to eradicate *H. pylori*, detecting almost immediately when the bacteria have been killed. With the blood test, *H. pylori* antibodies may still be present a year or more after the infection is gone.

Stool antigen test. This newer test checks for *H. pylori* in stool samples. It's useful in helping to diagnose *H. pylori* infection. It also may be useful in monitoring the success of treatment.

A combination of medications

An ulcer isn't something you should treat on your own, without a doctor's help. Over-the-counter antacids and acid blockers may relieve the gnawing pain, but the relief is always short-lived.

With a doctor's help, you can find prompt relief from ulcer pain as well as a lifelong cure from the disease. Because most ulcers stem from *H. pylori* bacteria, doctors use a two-pronged approach:
- Kill the bacteria.
- Reduce the level of acid in your digestive system to relieve pain and encourage healing.

Accomplishing these two steps requires use of at least two, and sometimes three or four, of the following types of medications.

Antibiotics

Several combinations of antibiotics kill *H. pylori*. Most of the medications are equally effective and destroy the bacteria in more than 90 percent of cases. However, for the treatment to work, it's essential that you follow your doctor's instructions precisely.

Antibiotics most commonly prescribed for treatment of *H. pylori* include amoxicillin (Amoxil), clarithromycin (Biaxin), metronidazole (Flagyl) and tetracycline (Achromycin). Some pharmaceutical companies package a combination of two antibiotics together, with an acid suppressor or cytoprotective agent specifically for treatment of *H. pylori* infection. These combination treatments are sold under the names Prevpac and Helidac.

You'll need to take antibiotics for only one to two weeks, depending on the type and number of antibiotics your doctor prescribes. Other medications prescribed in conjunction with antibiotics generally are taken for a longer period.

Acid blockers

Acid blockers — also called histamine (H-2) blockers — reduce the amount of hydrochloric acid released into your digestive tract to relieve ulcer pain and encourage healing. Normally, this acid isn't damaging to your stomach and duodenum. But if a defect develops in the mucous layer that coats your digestive tract, hydrochloric acid can seep into the defect and produce an ulcer. Other ulcer-promoting factors, including use of nicotine, NSAIDs and alcohol, increase the risk of the defect turning into an ulcer.

Acid blockers work by keeping histamine from reaching histamine receptors. Histamine is a substance normally present in your body. When it reacts with histamine receptors, the receptors signal acid-secreting cells in your stomach to release hydrochloric acid.

Available by prescription or over the counter, acid blockers include the medications cimetidine (Tagamet), famotidine (Pepcid), nizatidine (Axid) and ranitidine (Zantac). For treatment of ulcers, prescription acid blockers are more effective because they're stronger than over-the-counter products.

Antacids

Your doctor may include an antacid in your drug regimen. An antacid may be taken in addition to an acid blocker or in place of one. Instead of reducing acid secretion, antacids neutralize existing stomach acid and can provide rapid pain relief.

Proton pump inhibitors (PPIs)

A more effective way to reduce stomach acid is to shut down the pumps within acid-secreting cells. Proton pump inhibitors (PPIs) reduce acid by blocking the action of these tiny pumps. They include the prescription medications esomeprazole (Nexium), lansoprazole (Prevacid) and rabeprazole (Aciphex), and the over-the-counter medication omeprazole (Prilosec). Another drug, pantoprazole (Protonix), can be taken orally or received intravenously in the hospital. PPIs

Ulcers that fail to heal

Approximately 90 percent of all peptic ulcers heal within six to eight weeks. Those that don't are called refractory ulcers. There are many reasons why an ulcer may fail to heal. Not taking medications according to direction is one reason. Another is that some types of *H. pylori* are resistant to antibiotics. Other factors that can interfere with the healing process include regular use of tobacco, alcohol or NSAIDs. Sometimes the problem is accidental. People are unaware that a medication they're taking contains an NSAID.

In rare cases, refractory ulcers may be a result of extreme overproduction of stomach acid, an infection other than *H. pylori*, or other digestive diseases, including Crohn's disease or cancer.

Treatment for refractory ulcers generally involves eliminating factors that may interfere with healing, along with stronger doses of ulcer medications. Sometimes, additional medications may be included. Surgery to help heal an ulcer may be necessary only when the ulcer doesn't respond to aggressive drug treatment.

also appear to inhibit *H. pylori*. However, these drugs cost almost twice as much as acid blockers. Uncommon side effects include stomach pain, diarrhea and headache.

Cytoprotective agents

These medications are designed to help protect the tissues that line the stomach and small intestine. They include the prescription medications sucralfate (Carafate) and misoprostol (Cytotec). The drugs carry some side effects. Sucralfate may cause constipation. Misoprostol may cause diarrhea and uterine bleeding. Misoprostol shouldn't be taken by pregnant women because it can cause miscarriage.

Another cytoprotective agent is bismuth subsalicylate (Pepto-Bismol). In addition to protecting the lining of your stomach and intestines, bismuth preparations appear to inhibit *H. pylori* activity.

What you can do

Before the discovery of *H. pylori*, people with ulcers were often placed on a restricted diet and told to reduce the amount of stress in their lives. Now that food and stress have been eliminated as causes of ulcers, these factors no longer apply. However, while an ulcer is healing, it's still advisable to watch what you eat and control stress. Acidic or spicy foods may increase ulcer pain. The same is true for stress. Stress slows digestion, allowing food and digestive acid to remain in your stomach and intestines for a longer period.

Your doctor also may suggest these steps:
- Don't smoke.
- Avoid alcohol.
- To relieve pain, take acetaminophen (Tylenol, others) instead of NSAIDs.

If acetaminophen isn't effective, COX-2 inhibitors may be helpful. These prescription medications are designed to relieve muscle and joint pain without causing as many digestive problems. However, COX-2 inhibitors have been linked to serious health problems. Your doctor can advise you about the risks and benefits of COX-2s.

Nonulcer dyspepsia

Sometimes, people will see their doctors for what they think is an ulcer, but isn't. Although they may have gnawing upper abdominal pain, diagnostic tests don't reveal an ulcer or other digestive problem — all test results come back normal. Many of these people have nonulcer dyspepsia (dis-PEP-se-uh), from the Greek roots *dys,* meaning "difficult," and *peptein,* which means "to digest."

Nonulcer dyspepsia occurs for no apparent reason. Its most common symptom is pain, or an uncomfortable feeling, in your upper abdomen. As with an ulcer, the pain is often relieved with food or antacids. Other symptoms may include gas, bloating, nausea or feeling full after eating only a moderate amount.

Plenty of theories, little proof

The cause of nonulcer dyspepsia is largely unknown. It's possible the pain may stem from an irritation to your stomach lining. Researchers have other theories as well.

Presence of *H. pylori* bacteria. Your symptoms may represent an early case of *H. pylori* infection, even though you don't have an ulcer.

Reaction to drugs and supplements. Pain relievers such as aspirin and other NSAIDs are known to cause ulcers and gastritis. It's possible these medications may also irritate your digestive system without producing stomach or intestinal damage. The same may be true for other drugs and supplements, including antibiotics, steroids, minerals and herbs.

Overproduction of stomach acid. Acid-secreting cells in the stomach may produce higher than normal amounts of digestive acid. The oversupply may irritate digestive tissues.

Stomach disorder. For unknown reasons, your stomach may not function or empty normally. This sometimes happens after certain viral infections.

Acid sensitivity. Digestive tissues in the stomach and duodenum may be overly sensitive to normal acid levels and become easily irritated.

Food sensitivity. Your stomach or intestines may be overly sensitive to certain foods or food ingredients. Often, but not always, these include certain spices, citrus fruits or vegetables that contain moderate to high levels of acid. Some people also find that coffee seems to worsen symptoms.

Overreaction to normal stimuli. Nerve signals between your stomach and brain may be flawed, causing an exaggerated response to normal changes that take place during digestion, such as stretching of your stomach as it fills with food.

Stress. The pain may be your body's way of responding to stress.

Psychological disorder. Depression, anxiety or some other factor affecting your emotional health may play a role.

Lifestyle changes often first step

Symptoms of nonulcer dyspepsia are usually mild, and often the condition is treated by examining and changing daily habits. This may include avoiding foods that seem to worsen symptoms, controlling stress, and changing or limiting daily medications or supplements. Some people find that eating smaller but more frequent meals and low-fat foods also improves their symptoms.

If these practices don't help, your doctor may recommend drug therapy. Many of the same drugs used to treat ulcers are recommended for nonulcer dyspepsia, even, at times, antibiotics. Some people with nonulcer dyspepsia test positive for *H. pylori*. They don't have ulcers, but they do carry the bacteria that sometimes cause ulcers. Eradicating the bacteria, however, may not improve your symptoms.

Other therapies that may be helpful include the following.

Pain relievers. Drugs that block pain or its perception, including a low-dose antidepressant, may help desensitize digestive nerves. Antidepressants often work well for irritable bowel syndrome, which some researchers believe may be associated with nonulcer dyspepsia. However, further study is needed to determine the value of antidepressant therapy.

Antispasmodic drugs. These include the prescription medications dicyclomine (Bentyl) and hyoscyamine (Levsin). They're often effective at stopping muscle spasms in your digestive tract, but they haven't shown much promise in treating nonulcer dyspepsia.

Behavior therapy. If your doctor believes your condition may be related to stress or a psychological disorder, he or she may recommend that you see a psychiatrist, psychologist or nurse counselor. These health care professionals can help you develop ways to control stress or deal with other matters in your life that may be contributing to your symptoms.

Chapter 7

Irritable bowel syndrome

Y ou're out with friends, and you've just finished a delicious meal when the familiar rumblings in your stomach begin. You excuse yourself and head for home, where you spend the next hour suffering through cramps and diarrhea. Other times, you may battle uncomfortable constipation. Either way, your life at home and in the workplace suffers.

Key signs and symptoms
- Abdominal pain or discomfort
- Bloating or gas
- Diarrhea
- Constipation
- Mucus in stool

Irritable bowel syndrome (IBS) is a common problem that affects about one in five adults in the United States, most commonly women. IBS is sometimes called spastic colon because for years spasm of intestinal walls was thought to cause its symptoms. The walls of your intestines are lined with layers of muscle that contract and relax, helping to move food from your stomach, through your intestines to your rectum. Normally, the muscles contract and relax in coordinated rhythm. With IBS, they function abnormally. They contract for a longer time, and with more force than normal, causing pain. Food is forced through the intestines more quickly, producing gas, bloating and diarrhea. Sometimes, the opposite occurs. Passage of food and waste slows, leading to hard, dry stools.

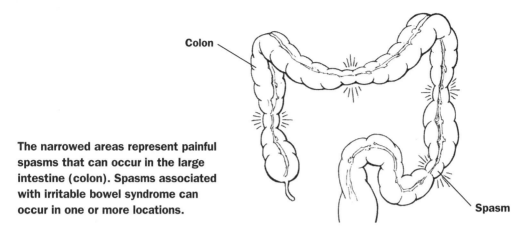

Colon

Spasm

The narrowed areas represent painful spasms that can occur in the large intestine (colon). Spasms associated with irritable bowel syndrome can occur in one or more locations.

Though IBS isn't life-threatening, it can interfere with your quality of life. If you have a mild form, the condition may be only a minor inconvenience. At the other end of the scale, the pain and accompanying symptoms can seem unbearable. Most people have mild symptoms. Some people have moderate symptoms that are intermittent but can be disabling. A small fraction of people with IBS have severe symptoms.

A functional disorder

IBS is often referred to as a functional disorder, meaning that your intestines look normal, but they function abnormally. No one knows for certain what causes IBS. Some researchers believe that the condition is related to nerves in the intestines that control sensation. These nerves may be more sensitive than normal, causing you to react strongly to certain foods, physical activity, or the presence of air or gas in your intestines. Something that might not bother most people, such as a little gas, may cause you pain or bloating.

Researchers also feel that stress and other psychological factors contribute to IBS. Many people find that their symptoms are more severe or frequent during stressful events, such as a change in their daily routine, family troubles or while attending social gatherings. For years, doctors attributed IBS to stress alone. But studies suggest both a functional (physiological) and an emotional (psychological) basis for IBS.

Because women are twice as likely as men to have IBS, researchers have speculated that hormonal changes may play a role. IBS may also result from another illness. Some people first experience IBS after an acute episode of diarrhea. However, IBS is not related to inflammatory bowel diseases such as Crohn's disease or ulcerative colitis. IBS also doesn't cause cancer or make you more likely to have cancer. IBS does run in families, and researchers are investigating the genetic component of the condition.

Ruling out other conditions

There isn't any test that can tell if you have IBS. Typically, the disorder is diagnosed when other conditions that can produce similar symptoms have been ruled out. Tests to exclude other conditions may include blood, stool and urine tests, X-rays, colonoscopy and transit studies. (See Chapter 4 for information about these tests.)

Your doctor also may ask about your psychological health. Do you feel stressed? How well do you cope with stress? Do you often feel depressed or anxious?

Before IBS is diagnosed, certain signs and symptoms — known as Rome criteria — must be present. The most important are abdominal pain and diarrhea or constipation that has occurred in at least 12 weeks out of the previous 12 months. At least two additional signs and symptoms that must be present at least 25 percent of the time to support a diagnosis of IBS include:

- Having a bowel movement more or less often than usual (more than three a day or less than three a week)
- Alternating hard and soft stools
- Straining to pass stools, urgent stools, or feeling that you can't empty your bowels completely
- Passing mucus in your stools
- Feeling bloated, or having abdominal swelling

Improving symptoms with diet and exercise

Because there isn't a cure for IBS, the focus of treatment is on managing your symptoms so that you can participate in normal activities and fully enjoy life. Treatment often is twofold:

- Identify factors that trigger your symptoms.

• Develop strategies to minimize your symptoms.

A healthy diet and regular exercise are good starting points. They can keep your digestive system functioning smoothly, reducing IBS symptoms. Keep in mind, however, that your body may not respond immediately to changes in your daily habits. Instead, look for signs of gradual improvement. Your goal is to find long-term, not temporary, solutions.

Eat low-fat foods

Fat stimulates contractions of the large intestine (colon), aggravating IBS symptoms. You don't need to avoid all fat, but if fat seems to worsen pain and diarrhea, limit the amount you eat. The best way to reduce fat in your diet is to eat more plant-based foods. Plant foods — fruits, vegetables and foods made from whole grains — contain beneficial vitamins, minerals, cancer-preventing compounds (phytochemicals) and fiber.

Experiment with fiber

For people with IBS, dietary fiber can be either good or bad. High-fiber foods soften and speed passage of stool, reducing constipation.

Is it IBS, or lactose or sorbitol intolerance?

If your cramping and bloating occur mainly after eating dairy products or sugar-free gum or candies, your problem may not be irritable bowel syndrome but another condition.

People with lactose intolerance have difficulty digesting the sugar (lactose) in dairy products because their bodies don't produce enough of the enzyme lactase. Lactase breaks down lactose so that it can be absorbed in your small intestine. When lactose isn't absorbed, it can cause cramping and diarrhea.

The artificial sweetener sorbitol found in some gums and candies also can produce symptoms similar to those of IBS. If cramping and abdominal pain typically occur from chewing sugar-free gum or eating sugar-free candy, your problem could simply be an intolerance to sorbitol.

But in some people, fiber worsens diarrhea, gas and pain. It may be that some with IBS are more sensitive to gases produced in the colon from fermentation of fiber.

The best approach is to gradually increase the amount of fiber in your diet over a period of weeks. If you continue to experience pain and diarrhea, talk with a dietitian about designing a low-fat diet that also includes reduced amounts of dietary fiber.

For more information on the types and amounts of food to eat regularly for good health, including foods highest in fiber, see Chapter 2.

Drink plenty of liquids

Liquids can help relieve constipation and replace body fluids absorbed by fiber. Each day drink at least eight glasses of fluids. Water is best. Beverages containing caffeine and alcohol cause you to urinate more. They can also worsen diarrhea by stimulating or irritating your intestines. Avoid carbonated beverages because they can produce gas.

Avoid problem foods

If you find that certain foods aggravate your symptoms, don't eat them. Many people with IBS notice an improvement in symptoms simply by excluding certain foods or beverages from their diets. Common culprits are fatty foods, beans and other gas-producing foods, alcohol and caffeine.

Eat at regular times

Don't skip meals, and try to eat at about the same time each day. Scheduled meals help regulate bowel function and lessen symptoms of constipation and diarrhea. That's because digestion stimulates the muscles in your colon to contract and move stool onward.

Some people find that eating frequent, smaller meals agrees with them better than eating three large meals a day. For others, especially people bothered by constipation, the opposite is true. To stimulate muscle contractions and passage of stool, they need to eat medium-sized to large meals.

Get active

Physical activity helps decrease feelings of stress. It also stimulates the rhythmic contractions of your intestines, helping them to function normally. Physical activity can relieve constipation and may alleviate symptoms of diarrhea. It can also improve depression and make you feel better about yourself.

Aim for 30 to 60 minutes of moderate physical activity most days of the week. If you've been inactive, begin slowly, and gradually increase the amount of time you exercise. For information on various types of exercise, see "Get regular exercise" on page 24.

Other helpful hints

These steps also may help relieve some of your symptoms:
- Soak in a warm bath or lie down with a hot-water bottle or heating pad on your abdomen to decrease abdominal pain. Be careful, however, not to burn your skin.
- Wear comfortable, loosefitting clothing so as not to put pressure on your abdomen.
- Go to the bathroom as soon as you feel the urge, but don't hurry yourself. Allow adequate time for a bowel movement without straining.

Learning to manage stress

Anyone can experience digestive upset from worry, anxiety or other stressful emotions. But in people with IBS, stress-related symptoms such as abdominal pain and diarrhea tend to occur more frequently and severely. A vicious cycle can develop. Your signs and symptoms can increase your stress level, which causes them to worsen, which further increases your stress, and so on.

Another important step in controlling IBS is learning how to relax. There are many methods of relaxation. Some people relax while listening to or performing music, or surrounding themselves with soothing aromas (aromatherapy). Others benefit from massage, yoga or meditation. Studies show that hypnosis also may reduce abdominal pain and bloating. A trained professional teaches you how to enter a relaxed (hypnotic) state and guides you through an imagery session during which you imagine your bowel muscles smooth, calm and still.

To help you get started, here are two simple relaxation techniques you can use when you begin to feel stressed.

Deep breathing. Most adults breathe from their chests. Each time you breathe in (inhale), your chest expands. Each time you breathe out (exhale), it contracts. To relax, breathe deeply from your diaphragm, the muscle that separates the chest from the abdomen. You can use deep breathing as your only means of relaxation or as a warm-up and cool-down method for other techniques (see "Taking a breather").

Progressive muscle relaxation. This technique involves relaxing a series of muscles one at a time. First, raise the tension level in a group of muscles, such as a leg or an arm, by tightening muscles and then relaxing them. Concentrate on slowly letting the tension go in each muscle. Then move on to the next muscle group.

Taking a breather

Here's an exercise to help you practice deep, relaxed breathing. Rehearse it throughout the day until you can automatically apply it when you feel stressed:

1. Sit comfortably with your feet flat on the floor.
2. Loosen tight clothing around your abdomen and waist.
3. Place your hands on your lap or at your sides.
4. Close your eyes if it helps you to relax.
5. Breathe in slowly through your nose while counting to four. Allow your abdomen to expand as you breathe in.
6. Pause for a second and then exhale at a normal rate through your mouth.
7. Repeat until you feel more relaxed.

Using over-the-counter medications

Nonprescription medications can help relieve your discomfort while you're taking steps to change your lifestyle. Depending on your symptoms, you may benefit from a nonprescription product.

Antidiarrheals

Loperamide (Imodium) slows the rate at which food leaves your intestines and increases intestinal water and ion (sodium) absorption, to help solidify stool. Other antidiarrheals, such as bismuth (Pepto-Bismol), also may relieve diarrhea and the urgency to have a bowel movement. You need to be careful, however, not to use antidiarrheal medications too often or too long. Overuse can lead to or worsen constipation. One approach is to take an antidiarrheal after each loose bowel movement. That way, the amount of treatment can match the severity of the diarrhea. Some people with IBS take an antidiarrheal before they go out to eat, to serve as a safety net and to avoid embarrassment.

You might also experiment with peppermint tea (tea that contains peppermint oil). There's some evidence it helps relieve diarrhea or gas accompanied by bloating. However, peppermint can aggravate heartburn.

Fiber supplements and laxatives

To relieve constipation, begin with a natural fiber supplement such as Metamucil or Citrucel. They should help within one to three days. When taken regularly as directed, fiber supplements are generally safe and effective. Because they're so absorbent, take them with plenty of water. Otherwise, they can become constipating — the opposite of what you want. If these measures don't help, ask your doctor about a laxative. There are several types.

Stool softeners. Sold over the counter under several brand names, these include Colace and Surfak. These are the most gentle products.

Avoid taking mineral oil to help soften your stools and relieve constipation. It can block absorption of key vitamins.

Saline laxatives. These are relatively safe to use long term and include the over-the-counter product Phillips' Milk of Magnesia. It works by increasing water content in your stool.

Stimulant laxatives. The most powerful of laxatives, these products may be considered when other measures fail to induce a bowel movement and after discussing their use with your doctor. Over-the-counter brand names include Dulcolax, Ex-Lax and Senokot.

Avoid the long-term, unsupervised use of laxatives. Talk with your doctor about the best use of these over-the-counter medications.

Medical treatment for more severe symptoms

If your symptoms are moderate to severe, you may need more help than lifestyle changes or over-the-counter medications can offer.

Prescription medications

Depending on your symptoms, your doctor may recommend one of the following medications.

Smooth-muscle relaxants. Anticholinergic (antispasmodic) drugs, such as hyoscyamine (Levsin) and dicyclomine (Bentyl), may help relax intestinal muscles and relieve muscle spasms. The medications have side effects including urinary retention, accelerated heart rate, blurred vision and dry mouth.

Antidepressants. These medications may be useful in treating IBS even if you're not depressed. In addition to treating depression, the drugs help relieve abdominal pain and diarrhea or constipation. Your doctor may recommend a tricyclic antidepressant or a selective serotonin reuptake inhibitor (SSRI).

The tricyclic agents amitriptyline (Elavil), imipramine (Tofranil), doxepin (Sinequan) and nortriptyline (Pamelor) are most frequently prescribed for abdominal pain especially if accompanied by diarrhea. Tricyclic antidepressants may cause drowsiness, dry mouth and constipation.

The SSRIs fluoxetine (Prozac) and paroxetine (Paxil) are recommended for abdominal pain. However, in some people SSRIs can cause nausea, cramping and diarrhea.

Antidepressants must be taken regularly to be effective. Because of this, these medications generally are prescribed only if you have chronic or recurring symptoms.

Alosetron (Lotronex). This medication was produced specifically for the treatment of IBS in women. The drug is especially useful for controlling diarrhea associated with the condition. Alosetron relaxes the large intestine and slows movement of waste through the large intestine. But some people taking the medication have experienced obstructed or ruptured bowels from complications of severe constipation or intestinal damage from reduced blood flow to the large intestine (ischemic colitis). Because of these severe side effects, the drug was withdrawn from the market for safety concerns in 2000. It was re-approved by the Food and Drug Administration in 2002 for use on a very restricted basis.

5-HT agonist agents. These medications are being developed to stimulate movement of waste through the colon and are used to treat constipation and abdominal pain. Tegaserod, a 5-HT-4 partial agonist agent, has been shown to help relieve abdominal pain, bloating and constipation in women with IBS.

Counseling

This is an important part of treatment if your condition is related to stress or anxiety. A health care professional who specializes in behavioral medicine, such as a psychiatrist or psychologist, can help you reduce stress and anxiety by examining your responses to life events, and then helping you to modify those responses. You learn to identify stressful situations that cause your bowel reactions and you develop strategies for dealing with the stress. For most people, counseling combined with medication works better than medication alone.

Chapter 8

Crohn's disease and ulcerative colitis

Crohn's disease and ulcerative colitis are digestive diseases that can be painful and debilitating. At their core is chronic diarrhea. Some people experience just a couple of episodes of diarrhea daily, others more than a half dozen. Among people with severe digestive disease, daily life revolves around a continual need to hurry to the bathroom, with the constant fear of an accident.

Key signs and symptoms

- Diarrhea
- Abdominal pain and cramping
- Blood in stool
- Fatigue
- Reduced appetite
- Weight loss
- Fever

Crohn's disease and ulcerative colitis are the two most common forms of inflammatory bowel disease, an umbrella term for inflammatory conditions that damage the digestive tract. There is no cure for Crohn's disease, named after Burrill Crohn, M.D., who, along with his colleagues, described the disease in 1932. The only cure for ulcerative colitis is surgical removal of the colon and rectum.

But there is good news. Although these diseases often can't be cured, they can be treated. There are several therapies that can drastically reduce your signs and symptoms, and possibly even bring about a long-term remission.

Similar but different

Crohn's disease and ulcerative colitis can behave so similarly that one is sometimes mistaken for the other. The two conditions share many of the same signs and symptoms. Both inflame the lining inside the digestive tract. Both can take an uncertain course, such as long-term flare-ups followed by periods of remission. And both may require a complex plan of drug therapy. In fact, the medications used to treat the diseases are often nearly identical.

Despite these similarities, the two have key differences. Crohn's disease can occur anywhere in your digestive tract, from your mouth to your anus. The inflammation can occur simultaneously in different locations, and it generally spreads deep through every layer of tissue in the affected areas.

Ulcerative colitis is limited to the colon and rectum. The inflammation often begins in the rectum and spreads continuously into the colon. The disease also differs from Crohn's in that only the innermost lining (mucosa) is affected. The inflammation typically doesn't involve deep tissues.

Though Crohn's disease and ulcerative colitis can occur at any age, the diseases often affect people between the ages of 15 and 35 and people between 50 and 80. Men and women are equally susceptible. Whites have the highest risk of inflammatory bowel disease, but the disease occurs in many ethnic groups. In particular, Jewish people of European descent are five times more likely to have inflammatory bowel disease than are other whites.

Crohn's disease and ulcerative colitis affect approximately 1 million Americans, with each condition accounting for roughly half that number. Some estimates are twice this high. The wide variation is partly because the diseases can be difficult to diagnose and many people don't realize they're affected.

In search of a cause

Though researchers haven't unlocked the mystery behind what causes these two diseases, there's a general consensus as to what doesn't cause them. Contrary to past belief, researchers no longer think that stress is a culprit, although it may aggravate symptoms. Nor do they think the diseases are passed on by infection from one person to another. As for what may trigger them, there are only theories.

Immune system. One theory is that the diseases are linked to an unknown virus or bacteria. The inflammation results from your body's immune system trying to fight off the invaders. In fact, drugs that suppress the immune system are proving remarkably effective in controlling signs and symptoms in many people. It's also possible that the inflammation may stem from the virus or the bacterium itself.

Heredity. Fifteen percent to 30 percent of people with Crohn's disease or ulcerative colitis have an immediate family member — a parent, a brother, a sister or a child — with an inflammatory bowel disease. Multiple genetic factors may make a person susceptible to inflammatory bowel disease. The details of these factors are the subject of intensive research.

Environment. Both diseases are more prevalent in developed nations and in cities. This has led some experts to speculate that environmental factors, such as diet, may play a role. Another theory is that people living in nations with cleaner environments may in essence be victims of good hygiene and public health measures. As a result, they're vulnerable to infections later in life, causing their immune systems to overreact.

Troublesome signs and symptoms

Each disease produces a variety of signs and symptoms. These may develop gradually or appear suddenly.

Crohn's disease
One or more of these signs or symptoms may occur and be mild to severe.

Diarrhea. Your intestines respond to the inflammation as they would to an infection. Intestinal cells may secrete additional salt and water. This process overwhelms the capacity of your lower small intestine and colon to absorb fluid. The muscles in your intestines may contract more often than normal. The result is diarrhea.

Cramping and vomiting. Persistent inflammation can cause scar tissue to form, which in turn can lead to the swelling and thickening of intestinal walls. Intestinal passageways may narrow, blocking the passage of waste. Cramping and vomiting can result.

Bleeding. As food waste passes through your digestive system and touches inflamed tissue, the tissue may bleed. Inflamed tissue may also bleed on its own, without the presence of food waste. The blood is expelled with your stool. It may be bright red and appear in the toilet bowl or dark in color and mixed with stool.

Weight loss and fatigue. If the inflammation is in your small intestine, where food nutrients are absorbed, you may not be able to absorb enough nutrients to maintain your weight and energy level. So you lose weight and tire easily. Excessive blood loss also can produce fatigue.

Malabsorption of nutrients may be the reason that children with Crohn's disease tend to have stunted growth. Young people ages 10 through 19 account for approximately 30 percent of people with inflammatory bowel disease. Two percent of cases involve children below age 10.

Ulcers. Chronic inflammation can produce an open sore (ulcer) anywhere in your digestive tract, even your mouth, esophagus or anus. Some people have a string of disconnected ulcers scattered throughout their digestive tracts. Typically, Crohn's-related ulcers develop in the lower small intestine (terminal ileum), colon, rectum or a combination of these.

Fistulas. Deep ulcers may burrow completely through the intestinal wall and create a fistula — an abnormal, tubular connection between internal organs or between an organ and the skin surface. Often, fistulas connect one loop of the small intestine to another. When a fistula develops between the small intestine and colon, food particles can take a shortcut through the opening and arrive in the colon before nutrients from the particles have been absorbed in the small intestine.

Sometimes, fistulas can develop into pockets of infection (abcesses), which can become life-threatening if left untreated. Treatment may involve medication or surgery, depending on the severity and location of the fistula.

Other complications. Crohn's disease can cause additional signs and symptoms and diseases, including:

- Inflammation, swelling, stiffness and pain in your joints
- Skin rashes or sores
- Anal skin tags, mimicking hemorrhoids
- Inflammation of your eyes
- Kidney stones
- Gallstones

It's uncertain what causes these problems. Some researchers believe they're linked to an immune system response that produces inflammation in parts of your body beyond the digestive tract. When the disease is treated, some signs and symptoms will disappear.

Is your disease mild, moderate or severe?

Mild Crohn's disease
- Four or fewer diarrheal bowel movements daily
- Minimal or no abdominal pain
- Healthy weight
- Few, if any, additional complications
- Normal temperature, pulse and red blood count

Moderate Crohn's disease
- Four to six diarrheal bowel movements daily
- Moderate abdominal pain
- Additional complications

Severe Crohn's disease
- Six or more diarrheal bowel movements daily
- Severe abdominal pain
- Underweight
- Additional complications
- Fever, rapid pulse, low red blood cell count, high white blood cell count

---

Ulcerative colitis

Like Crohn's disease, ulcerative colitis can cause diarrhea, bleeding, cramping, abdominal pain and similar complications. However, ulcerative colitis is more often associated with liver disease instead of kidney stones, gallstones or anal skin tags. With ulcerative colitis, stool often is mixed with blood, in addition to mucus from the lining of the colon or pus from ulcerations.

Toxic megacolon is a serious complication of ulcerative colitis that occurs in 2 percent to 8 percent of cases. The inflamed colon becomes immobilized and unable to expel stool and gas, causing it to become distended. Signs and symptoms of toxic megacolon include abdominal pain and swelling, fever and weakness. You may also become groggy or disoriented. Left untreated, the colon can rupture, leading to peritonitis, a condition in which bacteria from the colon enters the abdominal cavity, causing inflammation and infection that can be fatal. A ruptured colon requires emergency surgery.

Is your disease mild, moderate or severe?

Mild ulcerative colitis

- Four or fewer diarrheal bowel movements daily
- Occasional blood in the stool
- Normal temperature, pulse and red blood count
- Few, if any, additional complications

Moderate ulcerative colitis

- Four to six diarrheal bowel movements daily
- Blood in stool fairly regularly
- Additional complications

Severe ulcerative colitis

- Six or more diarrheal bowel movements daily
- Frequent blood in the stool
- Tender abdomen
- Additional complications
- Fever, rapid pulse, low red blood cell count, high white blood cell count

Diagnosing inflammatory bowel disease

There is no simple test to diagnose either Crohn's disease or ulcerative colitis. Like many other digestive conditions, the diseases most often are diagnosed after all other probable causes are ruled out.

Tests that can help confirm Crohn's disease or ulcerative colitis include the following.

Blood tests. An abnormal sedimentation rate or C-reactive protein level may indicate inflammation. Two tests — perinuclear anti-neutrophilic cytoplasmic antibody (pANCA) and anti-saccharomyces cerevisiae antibody (ASCA) — can occasionally help diagnose inflammatory bowel disease. These tests are about 80 percent to 90 percent accurate.

X-rays. Images of your small and large intestines may detect ulceration, swelling or complications such as a stricture or fistula.

Colonoscopy. This is the most definitive test for diagnosing Crohn's disease or ulcerative colitis. A doctor inserts a flexible tube about the diameter of an index finger into your colon. The tube contains a small video camera that sends images to a TV monitor.

If you have inflamed tissue, your bowel walls will bleed easily when gently touched by the probe. A single, continuous area of inflammation suggests ulcerative colitis. Tissue that has normal sections between areas of inflammation suggests Crohn's disease.

During the test, your doctor may also retrieve tissue samples (biopsy) to be examined under a microscope. Granulomas in the samples can confirm Crohn's disease, but often they're not present. Granulomas are small collections of inflammatory cells that typically surround and try to destroy bacteria and other foreign bodies. Granulomas don't usually occur with ulcerative colitis.

Helpful medications

Medications can't cure inflammatory bowel disease, but they can effectively reduce signs and symptoms in most people. The main goal of drug therapy is to reduce inflammation in your intestines, because that's what triggers most of your signs and symptoms. Doctors use several categories of drugs that control inflammation in different ways. Some drugs work well for some people, but not for others. So it may take time to discover which drug or combination of drugs works best for you.

Anti-inflammatory drugs
Anti-inflammatory drugs are often a first step in medical treatment of inflammatory bowel disease.

Sulfasalazine. This medication has been commonly prescribed for mild to moderate Crohn's disease and ulcerative colitis since the 1940s. Sulfasalazine (Azulfidine) is often effective in reducing the signs and symptoms of either disease, and it can help prevent a relapse of ulcerative colitis. Yet the drug carries side effects, such as loss of appetite, nausea, vomiting, skin rashes and headache.

Mesalamine and olsalazine. More recently, doctors have been turning to mesalamine (Asacol, Pentasa, Rowasa) and olsalazine (Dipentum). These drugs work similarly to sulfasalazine, but they produce fewer side effects. Like sulfasalazine, mesalamine and olsalazine can be taken by mouth as tablets or administered rectally in the form of medicated enemas or suppositories.

Mesalamine enemas can relieve signs and symptoms in people with ulcerative colitis of the lower (sigmoid) colon and rectum. You administer the enema at night, while lying on your left side so that the medication can bathe the walls of your sigmoid colon and rectum. Treatment continues every night for four to eight weeks or until your intestinal lining has healed. The drawback of this therapy is that retaining the medication can be difficult if your colon is very active (contracting).

Corticosteroids. Steroids effectively reduce inflammation regardless of where the disease is located, but they can cause numerous side effects, including a puffy face, acne, excessive facial hair, night sweats, insomnia, irritability and hyperactivity. More serious side effects include high blood pressure, diabetes, osteoporosis, cataracts, glaucoma and increased risk of infection. In children, prolonged use of steroids can stunt growth.

Corticosteroids are prescribed mainly for moderate to severe inflammatory bowel disease that doesn't respond to other treatment. Some of the more commonly used steroids are prednisone, methylprednisolone and hydrocortisone. Newer and slower-acting steroids, such as budesonide (Entocort), are proving safer and more effective for mild to moderate Crohn's disease of the small intestine.

Corticosteroids can be taken by mouth or used rectally as a suppository, enema or foam. The most common way to take corticosteroids is in tablet form. Rectal preparations are generally recommended for mild to moderate ulcerative colitis in the sigmoid colon or rectum. Intravenous steroids may be given if your condition is serious enough to require hospitalization.

Immunosuppressants

Immunosuppressants also reduce inflammation, but in a different way. They target your immune system, which may be causing the inflammation or contributing to it. One theory as to the cause of inflammatory bowel disease is that your immune system over-reacts to an outside virus or bacterium. To destroy the foreign agent, your immune system releases chemicals. Over time, these chemicals may damage digestive tissues, causing inflammation. Immunosuppressive drugs relieve inflammatory bowel disease by interfering with your immune system's ability to release such chemicals.

Azathioprine and 6-mercaptopurine. These are the most widely used immunosuppressants for treatment of inflammatory bowel disease. It can take up to three months before these drugs begin to work. Exactly how they work remains unclear, but studies have found azathioprine (Imuran) and 6-mercaptopurine (6-MP) effective in reducing signs and symptoms of inflammatory bowel disease and healing fistulas from Crohn's disease.

Infliximab. Infliximab (Remicade) is an immunosuppressive drug that's been shown to be a short-term treatment of moderate to severe Crohn's disease. It's bioengineered to neutralize a natural protein called tumor necrosis factor that causes inflammation.

In clinical trials, between 65 percent and 80 percent of people with Crohn's who were treated with infliximab experienced an improvement. The drug also reduced the number of fistulas. However, its benefits appear to decrease over time. Because the drug is fairly new, its long-term safety also is uncertain.

Methotrexate. Long used to treat psoriasis and rheumatoid arthritis, in addition to cancer, this drug is sometimes recommended for people with Crohn's disease and ulcerative colitis who can't tolerate or don't respond well to other medications. Short-term side effects may include nausea. Long-term use of the drug may lead to scarring of the liver, but this is uncommon.

Cyclosporine. This potent drug is most often used in people who don't respond to other medications. The drug is beneficial for people with Crohn's disease who have fistulas. It also may improve signs and symptoms in people with severe ulcerative colitis.

However, cyclosporine can produce significant side effects. They include excessive hair growth, numbness of your hands and feet, seizures, high blood pressure, and liver and kidney damage.

Immunosuppressive therapy requires close monitoring by your doctor to avoid toxicity. Blood tests are done and medication dosages may need to be adjusted depending on the results.

Antibiotics

Antibiotics generally aren't effective for ulcerative colitis, but they can heal fistulas and abscesses and cause a remission of signs and symptoms in some people with Crohn's disease.

Metronidazole. This is one of the more commonly used antibiotics for Crohn's disease. Because it can cause serious side effects, how you take the drug is carefully regulated.

Side effects of metronidazole (Flagyl) can include numbness and tingling in your hands and feet and, sometimes, pain and muscle weakness. Reversal of the symptoms is slow, and they may never disappear. Other less serious side effects include nausea, headache, yeast infection and loss of appetite. In addition, the drug may cause a metallic taste. Hard candy or chewing gum can help mask the taste. Consuming alcohol while taking metronidazole can lead to severe side effects.

Ciprofloxacin. An alternative to metronidazole, ciprofloxacin (Cipro) is becoming the preferred choice. It improves signs and symptoms in 50 percent to 70 percent of certain people with Crohn's disease. Side effects include hypersensitivity to light and, in children, possible stunting of growth.

Others. Tetracycline or the combination of sulfamethoxazole and trimethoprim (Bactrim, Septra) may be taken for Crohn's disease. Side effects can include numbness and tingling in your hands and feet. Discontinuing these drugs too soon may cause a relapse, so long-term treatment is generally required.

Nicotine gum and patches

In clinical trials, nicotine gum and skin patches (the same kind that smokers use to help them quit) seem to provide short-term relief from flare-ups of ulcerative colitis. Nicotine supplied by gum or patch eliminates signs and symptoms in some people, but it appears to be effective only in the short run. After a while, signs and symptoms return in most people.

How nicotine works in easing inflammation isn't clear. Researchers suspect it may protect the colon by thickening and increasing the mucus that covers the lining where inflammation typically occurs. Nicotine may also reduce the actual inflammation.

Other medications

In addition to controlling inflammation, medications can help relieve your signs and symptoms. Your doctor may recommend that you take one or more of the following drugs, depending on your signs and symptoms.

Antidiarrheals. For mild to moderate diarrhea, a teaspoon of a fiber supplement (Metamucil, Citrucel) mixed with water twice a day may reduce diarrhea. Fiber adds bulk to stool as it absorbs water. For more severe diarrhea, loperamide (Imodium) or prescription narcotics can relax and slow the movement of your intestinal muscles. Narcotics, however, must be used with caution because they can produce side effects, including risk of toxic megacolon.

Laxatives. Narrowing of intestinal passages because of swelling can occasionally lead to constipation. Laxatives can help prevent constipation, but ask your doctor before taking any laxative. Even popular brands sold over the counter can be too harsh on your digestive system.

Pain relievers. For mild pain, your doctor may recommend acetaminophen (Tylenol). Avoid nonsteroidal anti-inflammatory drugs (NSAIDs). These include aspirin (Bayer, Bufferin), ibuprofen (Advil, Motrin, others), naproxen (Aleve) and ketoprofen (Orudis). Rather than reducing signs and symptoms of inflammatory bowel disease, they may aggravate them. One study found that people with ulcerative colitis who took NSAIDs doubled their risk for emergency treatment of a digestive-related problem. For moderate to severe pain, a prescription drug may be more effective.

Iron supplements. Blood loss from intestinal bleeding can cause iron deficiency anemia. Iron supplements restore adequate blood levels of iron and cure this type of anemia. The hormone erythropoietin is being tested for severe cases of anemia that don't respond to iron alone. Erythropoietin works in your bone marrow to increase the production of red blood cells.

Vitamin B-12 injections. Vitamin B-12 is absorbed in the terminal ileum, a portion of the small intestine commonly affected by Crohn's disease. If Crohn's is preventing absorption of this essential vitamin, you may need B-12 shots once a month for the rest of your life. People who have two or more feet of the terminal ileum removed during surgery also require lifelong B-12 injections.

Living with your disease

Long periods of remission are possible with both Crohn's disease and ulcerative colitis. But often the signs and symptoms return. In addition to medication, these steps can help control your signs and symptoms and lengthen the time between flare-ups.

Manage your diet

There's no firm evidence to suggest that the food you eat can cause or contribute to your disease. However, certain foods and beverages may aggravate your signs and symptoms, especially during a flare-up in your condition.

It's also important to understand that what applies to someone else may not apply to you. Some people with Crohn's disease or ulcerative colitis need to restrict their diet all of the time, others only some of the time, and still others never.

If you think that your diet is worsening your condition, experiment with different foods and beverages to see if eliminating some or adding others helps you feel better. Here are some steps to try.

Limit dairy products. Some people with Crohn's disease and ulcerative colitis have less diarrhea, pain and gas if they limit consumption of dairy products. These people may be lactose-intolerant. They aren't able to digest the milk sugar (lactose) in dairy products because they lack enough of the enzyme lactase. Lactase breaks down lactose into simple sugars that your body can absorb. If you find that dairy products seem to worsen your signs and symptoms, talk with a registered dietitian about designing a healthy diet that's low in lactose. For more information on lactose intolerance, see "Living with lactose intolerance" on page 36.

Restrict fiber. High-fiber foods, such as fruits, vegetables and grains, are the foundation of a healthy diet. But for some people with inflammatory bowel disease, fiber can have a laxative effect, worsening diarrhea. Fiber can also increase gas. Experiment with high-fiber foods to see if you're able to tolerate some better than others. If fiber remains a problem, you may have to restrict fruits, vegetables and grains in your diet. A dietitian can help you replace the nutrients these foods provide.

Reduce fat. People with severe Crohn's disease of the small intestine sometimes need to reduce fat in their diets because the small intestine is unable to absorb fat. Instead, fat passes through the intestine, causing or worsening diarrhea.

Reducing fat in your diet isn't a problem, unless you're unable to maintain a healthy weight. If you need to gain weight, talk with your doctor or a dietitian about how best to increase calories in your diet without increasing fat.

Ask about multivitamins. Because inflammatory bowel disease can interfere with normal absorption of nutrients, your doctor or dietitian may also suggest that you take a multivitamin that provides 100 percent of the Recommended Dietary Allowance (RDA) for essential vitamins and minerals. Individual vitamin, mineral or herbal supplements should be taken only under your doctor's supervision. They can interfere with your medication or you body's ability to absorb nutrients.

Drink plenty of fluids. Beverages offset fluid loss from diarrhea. Drink at least eight 8-ounce glasses of fluid, preferably water, daily. Avoid beverages that contain caffeine or alcohol, which promote urination and fluid loss.

Reduce stress

Stress doesn't cause inflammatory bowel disease, but it can worsen your signs and symptoms and may spark flare-ups. Many people with Crohn's disease or ulcerative colitis report increased digestive problems when they're under moderate to severe stress, such as when experiencing troubles at work, or after the death of a loved one.

During stress, your normal digestive process changes. Your stomach empties more slowly and acid-secreting cells release more juices. Stress can also speed or slow passage of food waste through your intestines, although much is still unknown about how stress affects the small and large intestines.

You can't avoid some forms of stress. But you can learn to manage ordinary daily stress with exercise, adequate rest and relaxation techniques, such as deep breathing, listening to relaxing music and meditation.

Seek information and support

Beyond the physical manifestations of Crohn's disease and ulcerative colititis, these diseases can cause emotional scars. Chronic diarrhea can lead to embarrassing accidents. Some people become so humiliated they begin to isolate themselves, rarely leaving home. When they do go out, their anxiety often makes their symptoms worse. Left untreated, these factors — isolation, humiliation and anxiety — can severely affect your life and lead to depression.

Many people with inflammatory bowel disease find emotional support simply by learning more about their disease and talking with their doctors or nurses. Schedule a time that you can discuss your fears and frustrations and ask questions about your condition. You might also consider joining a support group. Organizations such as the Crohn's and Colitis Foundation of America (CCFA) have chapters across the country. Your doctor, nurse or dietitian can help you locate the chapter nearest you or you can contact the organization for more information. (See "Additional resources" beginning on page 185.)

Some people find it helpful to consult a psychologist or psychiatrist about their anxieties. Try to find a professional who's familiar with inflammatory bowel disease and understands some of the emotional difficulties it causes.

Surgery

For most people with Crohn's disease or ulcerative colitis, drug therapy or changes in lifestyle don't offer significant improvement of their signs and symptoms. About 75 percent have surgery to treat their conditions.

With Crohn's disease, removal of a portion of your small or large intestine can provide years of relief. During the procedure, healthy sections of intestine are reconnected after the damaged portion is removed. The surgeon may also close fistulas and remove scar tissue that's blocking or narrowing the intestinal passageway. Newer laparoscopic surgical techniques require much smaller incisions than traditional surgery and allow for shorter recovery times.

But surgery often isn't a cure. The disease may come back, simply showing up elsewhere along your digestive tract.

Ulcerative colitis is different. Surgery can often cure the disease. Unfortunately, the procedure often entails removing your entire

Crohn's, colitis and colon cancer

Both ulcerative colitis and Crohn's disease can increase your risk of colon cancer. For ulcerative colitis, risk of colon cancer depends on how long you've had the disease and how much of your colon is affected. You're at increased risk of colon cancer if you've had ulcerative colitis for eight to 10 years and if the disease has spread through your entire colon. The smaller the area of the colon that's diseased, generally the lower the risk of cancer.

For Crohn's disease of the colon, how long you've had the disease and the extent of damage also are key factors. The longer you've had Crohn's disease and the larger the area of your colon that it covers, the greater your risk of colon cancer. Colon cancer, however, tends to be less common in people with Crohn's disease because, unlike ulcerative colitis, Crohn's disease often doesn't affect the entire colon. In addition, people with Crohn's disease are more likely to have surgery to remove the damaged portion of the colon.

If you've had inflammatory bowel disease of the colon for eight or more years, have a test for colon cancer every one to three years. The most effective test is colonoscopy.

colon and rectum. About 20 percent to 25 percent of people with ulcerative colitis undergo surgery because of continual bleeding, severe illness or risk of cancer.

Two variations

Surgery to remove the colon and rectum is call proctocolectomy (prok-toh-koh-LEK-tuh-me). Using the traditional approach to this surgery, an opening (stoma) about the size of a quarter is made in the lower right corner of the abdomen, near the beltline. After removal of the colon and rectum, the last portion of the small intestine (ileum) is attached to the stoma. A small bag (ileostomy bag) is worn over the stoma to collect waste, and periodic emptying of the bag is needed. This surgery is used mainly for older people who don't have good control of the anal sphincter muscle.

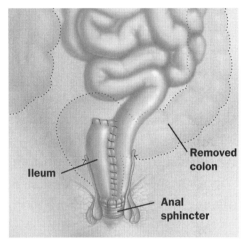

In ileoanal anastomosis, a surgeon removes the colon and innermost lining of the rectum, creates a J-shaped pouch out of the last section of the small intestine (ileum), then reattaches the pouch near the anal sphincter. Leaving the anal sphincter and rectal muscles intact allows near-normal passage of stool.

An alternative procedure used for most people eliminates the need to wear a bag. Called ileoanal anastomosis, this surgery takes advantage of the fact that inflammation associated with ulcerative colitis generally doesn't involve deep tissues. The surgeon removes your colon and the innermost lining of your rectum. A small J-shaped pouch is constructed from the end of your small intestine (ileum) and is attached directly to the anus and supported by remaining layers of rectal tissue. Waste is stored in the pouch and expelled normally, though bowel movements are more frequent and watery. You may have four to six loose bowel movements a day.

Ileoanal anastomosis surgery is usually done through a long incision across the midline of the abdomen. However, some specially trained surgeons perform this procedure laparoscopically, which helps to shorten hospital stays and recovery time.

Chapter 9

Celiac disease

It may have started with a viral infection, during pregnancy or while you were under a lot of stress. You kept experiencing intermittent diarrhea and bloating and you lost weight. But the signs and symptoms continued after the infection cleared up, the pregnancy was over or your stressful situation resolved itself. What may have happened is that your initial condition triggered a second one, called celiac disease — an intestinal disorder with lifelong implications.

Key signs and symptoms

- Diarrhea
- Abdominal gas and bloating
- Fatigue
- Weight loss
- Stunted growth (in children)
- Osteoporosis
- Anemia

Celiac disease damages the small intestine and interferes with its ability to absorb certain nutrients from food. People with celiac disease can't tolerate gluten, a protein found in wheat, barley and rye.

If you have celiac disease and you eat gluten, it causes an immune system reaction that inflames and swells the lining of the small intestine. The inflammation in turn causes tiny hairlike projections (villi) in the small intestine to shrink and even disappear. Villi (VIL-i) absorb vitamins, minerals and other nutrients in food. Without them, your body doesn't absorb necessary nutrients. Over time, poor absorption (malabsorption) of nutrients can deprive your brain, nervous system, bones, liver and other organs of nourishment, and cause vitamin deficiencies that can lead to illness.

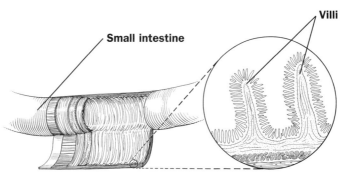

The inside of your small intestine is lined with tiny hairlike projections called villi. These projections increase the surface area of the small intestine, making it easier for the intestinal cells to absorb food nutrients.

An inherited condition

Also known as celiac sprue, nontropical sprue and gluten-sensitive enteropathy, celiac disease sometimes occurs in people who have an inherited inability to tolerate gluten. One large study has shown that if you have the disease, about 5 percent of your immediate blood relatives — brothers, sisters, parents, children — will likely have it as well.

Celiac disease affects about one in 200 people in the United States. It can occur at any age, and it tends to be more common in people of European descent and people with other autoimmune disorders, such as lupus erythematosus, type 1 diabetes (formerly called juvenile or insulin-dependent diabetes), rheumatoid arthritis or autoimmune thyroid disease. Some people first notice symptoms as children, others as adults. Many times, the disease emerges following some form of stress, such as an infection, pregnancy, physical injury or surgery. How or why these conditions may trigger celiac disease is unclear.

Varied signs and symptoms

Celiac disease may date back thousands of years, but it has only been in the last 50 years that researchers have gained a better understanding of the condition and how to treat it.

There is no typical form of the disease. Some people have no signs and symptoms and may live with celiac disease for years before it's diagnosed. Among people with signs and symptoms, they vary and may include fatigue, abdominal pain, intermittent diarrhea, bloating and excessive passing of gas. Fatigue stems from a reduction in red blood cells (anemia). Two other indications that nutrients are passing through your digestive tract without being absorbed are weight loss and lighter-colored, foul-smelling stools.

Celiac disease also may present itself in less obvious ways, including behavior changes such as irritability or depression, stomach upset, joint pain, muscle cramps, skin rash, mouth sores, dental and bone disorders, and tingling in your legs.

If you have celiac disease, you have higher-than-normal levels of antibodies to gluten circulating in your blood. Tests that measure anti-gliadin antibodies (AGA), anti-endomysial antibodies (EMA) and tissue transglutaminase antibodies (TTg) can detect celiac disease at an early stage. The test for TTg antibodies has proven particularly effective, identifying celiac disease in 98 percent of cases.

If blood tests and symptoms suggest celiac disease, your doctor may want to remove a tiny piece of tissue (biopsy) from your small intestine and examine it for damaged villi. The tissue is generally obtained by threading a thin, flexible tube (endoscope) through your mouth, esophagus and stomach into your small intestine.

Improvement in signs and symptoms after eliminating gluten from your diet also is a sign that you have celiac disease.

Similar but different diseases

Several conditions can cause malabsorption and may resemble celiac disease. They include tropical sprue, Whipple's disease, giardiasis infection, bacterial overgrowth and immunoglobulin deficiency. These conditions usually are distinguished from celiac disease by their special features. In addition, they don't respond to a gluten-free diet.

Dermatitis herpetiformis is an itchy, blistering skin disease that also stems from gluten intolerance. The rash usually occurs on the elbows, knees and buttocks. Dermatitis herpetiformis can cause significant intestinal damage identical to that of celiac disease. However, it may not produce noticeable digestive signs or symptoms. The disease is treated with a gluten-free diet, in addition to medication to control the rash.

However, don't go on a gluten-free diet before consulting your doctor. It can cause blood tests and biopsies to appear normal.

A new way of eating

There aren't any medications or surgeries that can cure celiac disease. The main treatment is a change in diet. To manage the disease and prevent complications, it's crucial that you avoid all foods that contain gluten. That means all foods or food ingredients made from most grains, including wheat, barley and rye. Whether people with celiac disease can safely eat oats is controversial. Recent studies have found that moderate amounts of oats had no harmful effects on intestinal mucosa. However, some experts continue to be concerned that oats contain amino acids that can be harmful.

At first, you also may need to take vitamin and mineral supplements recommended by your doctor or a dietitian to help correct nutritional deficiencies. As your condition and ability to absorb nutrients improve, your need for supplements may diminish. If you have osteoporosis due to celiac disease, you may need to continue taking calcium and vitamin D supplements long term.

Within just a few days after removing gluten from your diet, inflammation in your small intestine will likely begin to subside. It can take from several months to two to three years for your intestine to heal completely.

Getting used to your new diet can be difficult. Learning what foods you can and can't eat may take several months. You may crave foods that you're no longer allowed to eat. But don't give up. With time, most people learn to adjust to a gluten-free diet, and it becomes a normal part of their daily routines.

If you accidentally eat a product that contains gluten, you may or may not experience abdominal pain and diarrhea. Trace amounts of gluten in your diet still can be damaging. Over time, they can lead to complications, including anemia, osteoporosis, seizures, cancer and, in children, stunted growth. Going on and off a gluten-free diet also increases your risk of malnutrition and other complications, such as lymphoma and colon cancer.

Foods that contain gluten
Most foods made from grains contain gluten. Avoid these foods unless they're made with corn or rice or labeled as gluten-free.

- Breads
- Cereals
- Crackers
- Pasta
- Cookies
- Cakes and Pies
- Gravies
- Sauces

Food ingredients that contain gluten
Avoid all foods that include any of the following ingredients.

- Wheat (wheat flour, white flour, wheat bran, wheat germ, farina, wheat starch, graham flour, semolina, durum)
- Barley
- Rye
- Oats (oat flour, oat bran, oatmeal)
- Bulgur
- Kamut
- Kasha
- Matzo meal
- Spelt
- Triticale

New grain-containing products appear on the market periodically. Avoid them until you can verify their safety with a reliable source, such as a dietitian.

Other ingredients that may contain gluten
Because many processed foods have ingredients that contain gluten, it's important to check food labels. However, you can't always tell by reading the food label whether an ingredient is gluten-free. For example, hydrolyzed vegetable protein (HVP) may appear on the list of ingredients, but the label doesn't indicate

Sources of support
Many people can help you adjust to a gluten-free diet. Your doctor and a registered dietitian are first on the list. Your community may even have a support group for people with celiac disease. A number of national organizations also provide support services, including diet information. See "Additional resources" beginning on page 185.

whether HVP comes from soy, corn or wheat. Therefore, it's not safe, unless you know that it's made from soy or corn and not wheat. Avoid processed foods unless you can verify from the manufacturer that the ingredients don't contain gluten. (See "Reading food labels" on page 125.)

So what can you eat?

Though it may seem so, not all foods contain gluten. And with time and patience, you'll find many common foods you can still eat and enjoy. They include:

- Plain meats (not breaded or marinated)
- Fruits
- Vegetables
- Pasta from corn, rice and other gluten-free grains
- Quinoa
- Rice, including cereal and crackers made from rice
- Potatoes and potato flour
- Most dairy products
- Tapioca
- Amaranth
- Buckwheat

There are many gluten-free flours that you can use to make breads, cakes and other foods. Because even gluten-free grains can become contaminated with gluten-containing grains during harvest or processing, be sure that the label indicates that the flour is gluten-free, or

Hidden sources of gluten

You may ingest gluten in ways that you would never expect. One example is through cross contamination, when gluten-free foods come in contact with foods containing gluten. This may happen if you share a knife for spreading butter that has breadcrumbs on it, use the same toaster as others or eat deep-fried foods that are cooked in the same oil used for breaded foods.

Products other than food also may contain gluten, including:

- Medications that use gluten as a binding agent in a pill or tablet
- Lipstick
- Postage stamps

Your best bet is to contact the manufacturers of these products to find out if they contain gluten. In the case of stamps, use the self-adhesive kind.

that the manufacturer ensures that it is. You can also purchase ready-made gluten-free products. A dietitian can help you locate these products. Members of a local or national celiac disease support group also can be helpful in identifying foods that are safe to eat.

To assist you when shopping, some national support groups have published books or brochures that list manufactured and commercially produced grocery items that don't contain gluten. You can get copies of these shopping guides by contacting the Tri-County Celiac Sprue Support Group (TCCSSG) or Celiac Sprue Association (CSA). Addresses for these organizations are listed in "Additional resources" beginning on page 185. Make sure to use a guide that's been updated within the past two years.

Reading food labels

Food labels are important in making safe food choices. Always read the food label before you purchase any product. Some foods that seem acceptable, such as rice or corn cereals, may contain gluten. What's more, a manufacturer may change a product's ingredients at any time. A food that was once gluten-free no longer may be. Unless you read the label every time you shop, you won't know.

If you can't tell by the label if a food includes gluten, don't eat it until you get that information from a gluten-free shopper's guide or the product's manufacturer. It's a good idea to check with manufacturers periodically to be sure the information you have is current.

Eating out

Preparing your own meals is the best way to ensure your diet is gluten-free. But that doesn't mean that you can't eat out on occasion. The following guidelines can help you have a safe and enjoyable dining experience:

- Select a restaurant that specializes in the kinds of foods you can eat. You may want to call the restaurant in advance and discuss its menu options and your dietary needs.
- Visit the same restaurants so that you become familiar with their menus and the personnel get to know your needs.

- Ask members of your support group for suggestions on restaurants that serve gluten-free food.
- Follow the same practices you do at home. Select simply prepared or fresh foods and avoid all breaded or batter-coated foods.

Celiac disease and lactose intolerance

Because of damage to your small intestine from gluten, foods that don't contain gluten also may cause abdominal pain and diarrhea. Some people with celiac disease aren't able to tolerate milk sugar (lactose) found in dairy products, a condition called lactose intolerance. In addition to avoiding gluten, these people also need to limit food and drinks containing lactose.

Once your intestine has healed, you may be able to tolerate dairy products again. However, some people continue to experience lactose intolerance despite successful management of celiac disease. If you're among this group, you'll need to limit or avoid products that contain lactose for the rest of your life.

A dietitian can help you plan a diet that's low in lactose as well as gluten-free. If you can't eat dairy products, it's important that you include other sources of calcium in your diet.

When diet isn't enough

Approximately 70 percent of people with celiac disease who follow a gluten-free diet return to normal health within a few weeks. A small percentage who have severely damaged small intestines don't improve with a gluten-free diet. When diet isn't effective, treatment often includes medications to control intestinal inflammation and other conditions resulting from malabsorption. Because celiac disease is a lifelong condition, it's important to see your doctor regularly to be monitored for changes in your health.

Chapter 10

Diverticular disease

The general term for the development of small, bulging pouches in the digestive tract is *diverticular disease.* Each pouch is called a *diverticulum* (di-ver-TIK-yuh-lum), from Latin words meaning "a small diversion from the normal path." The name for more than one diverticulum is *diverticula.*

Key signs and symptoms

- Pain in the lower-left abdomen
- Abdominal tenderness
- Fever
- Nausea
- Constipation or diarrhea

Diverticula can form anywhere, including your throat, esophagus, stomach and small intestine. The most common site is your large intestine (colon), particularly the lower part of the colon called the sigmoid colon.

Diverticular disease is divided into two forms.

Diverticulosis

This condition refers to the formation of diverticula in the digestive tract. Diverticulosis is common and becomes more prevalent with advancing age. Nearly half the Americans older than age 60 have diverticula somewhere along their digestive tracts, most often in their colons. These pouches ordinarily don't cause any problems, and many people with the condition don't know they have it.

A minority of people with diverticulosis may experience mild abdominal cramps, bloating, gas, diarrhea or constipation. However, these signs and symptoms more likely are related to another condition, such as irritable bowel syndrome, and not diverticulosis. Bleeding isn't usually a sign of diverticulosis, but it can occur in some people (see "When a pouch bleeds" on page 129).

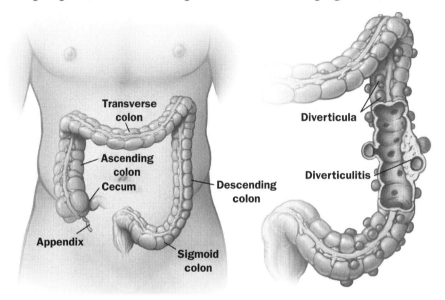

The most common location for small pouches (diverticula) is the large intestine (colon). When a pouch becomes inflamed or infected, the condition is called diverticulitis.

Diverticulitis

In a small percentage of people with diverticulosis, inflammation or an infection can develop in a diverticulum (diverticulitis). Some people experience only minor inflammation and others a massive, painful infection. One cause of diverticulitis is lodging of a small portion of stool in a pouch. The stool interrupts blood flow to the pouch and makes it susceptible to invasion of bacteria. A small tear also can develop in a diverticulum, leading to infection and, perhaps, a collection of pus (abscess).

Generally, the inflammation or infection is limited to the area directly around the diverticulum. In rare cases, the pouch can rupture, spilling intestinal waste into your abdominal cavity. This can lead to peritonitis (per-ih-to-NI-tis), an inflammation of the lining of the abdominal cavity. Peritonitis is a medical emergency demanding immediate attention.

Unlike diverticulosis, which generally causes no signs and symptoms, diverticulitis typically causes pain, fever and nausea. The pain often is abrupt and severe, but some people experience mild pain that gradually worsens over several days. Symptoms of diverticulitis are similar in many ways to those of appendicitis, except that the pain is usually in the lower-left side of your abdomen, instead of the lower right.

Less common signs and symptoms include vomiting, bloating, rectal bleeding, frequent urination, and difficulty or pain while urinating.

When a pouch bleeds

A small percentage of people with diverticulosis experience painless rectal bleeding. The blood may be dark and mixed with stool, or it may be red and visible in the toilet bowl. This bleeding may be the result of a weakened blood vessel in a diverticulum that has burst.

Bleeding from the ruptured blood vessel is typically shortlived. It often stops by itself, without treatment. If the bleeding is severe or persistent, you may need tests to identify the location of the bleeding. Occasionally, surgery to remove the segment of colon where the bleeding pouch is located is the only way to stop the bleeding.

A pressure problem

Why some people have diverticula and others don't isn't well understood. However, three factors seem to play a role.

Weak spots in colon wall

The colon is ringed by a layer of muscle that contracts repetitively to propel food waste to the rectum. Blood vessels penetrate the muscular ring to supply nutrients to the inner layer of the colon wall. The locations of the blood vessels are structurally weaker than the rest of the colon wall. When you strain to pass stool, increased pressure in your colon can cause these weak spots to bulge out.

Aging

Research suggests that as you age, the outer muscular wall of the colon thickens, causing the inside passageway to narrow. The narrowing increases pressure in your colon and the risk of pouch formation. Thickening of the outer wall also makes the colon less able to move food waste. The waste stays in the colon longer, where it exerts pressure on inner tissues.

Too little fiber

Diverticular disease emerged after the introduction of steel rolling mills into the flour milling process. This greatly reduced the fiber content of flour and other grain-derived foods. The disease was first observed in the United States in the early 1900s, around the time processed foods became a mainstay of the American diet. Diverticular disease is more common in industrialized nations, such as the United States, where the average diet is high in refined carbohydrates and low in fiber. In countries where people eat a high-fiber diet, diverticular disease is rare.

Too little fiber contributes to small, hard stools that are difficult to pass, increasing pressure in your colon. The highest pressures occur in the sigmoid colon, where most diverticula are found.

Accidental discovery

Because diverticula often don't cause problems, most people first learn they have diverticulosis during routine screening exams for colorectal cancer or during tests to determine the cause of intestinal symptoms. Colonoscopy, sigmoidoscopy, a computerized tomography (CT) scan or a colon X-ray may reveal one or more pouches.

Diverticulitis, on the other hand, is typically diagnosed while signs and symptoms such as abdominal pain, fever and nausea are present. Your doctor will examine your abdomen for tenderness. You also may receive a blood test to check your white blood cell count. An elevated number of white blood cells and tenderness in the lower-left abdomen may signal diverticulitis. Imaging tests such as a CT scan may help detect inflammation or infection of the colon. Diagnostic procedures are discussed in Chapter 4.

Treatment begins with self-care

How your condition is treated will depend on your signs and symptoms and whether the pouches are inflamed. If you don't have any signs and symptoms or they're mild, you may be able to treat the condition with changes in your daily habits. These same changes may also help prevent a second attack of diverticulitis.

The key to managing diverticular disease is to minimize the pressure inside your colon. To do that, follow these guidelines.

Eat more fiber
High-fiber foods, such as fresh fruits and vegetables and whole-grain products, soften stool and help it pass more quickly through the colon. This reduces pressure inside your digestive tract.

Depending on your age and sex, aim for 21 to 38 grams of fiber each day. (See "Where to find fiber" on page 15 for a list of high-fiber foods.) Try to substitute fruits, vegetables and grain products for foods high in fat.

People with mild signs and symptoms of diverticular disease often find that after a week or two of eating more fiber they begin to improve. However, avoid increasing the amount of fiber in your diet all at once. This can lead to uncomfortable gas, cramping, bloating and diarrhea. Gradually increasing fiber over a couple of weeks usually works best.

If you find it difficult to consume the recommended amount of fiber each day, talk with your doctor about regular use of a natural fiber supplement. These include over-the-counter products such as

Don't be afraid of seeds

You may have heard or read that eating foods containing seeds, such as those in raspberries or strawberries, is dangerous because the seeds can become lodged in a diverticulum and cause inflammation or infection.

This has never been shown to be true. You shouldn't forgo healthy fruits that contain seeds for fear of an infection. The fiber these foods provide outweighs the risk of diverticulitis.

psyllium (Metamucil) and methylcellulose (Citrucel). These products often relieve constipation within one to three days and can also help prevent constipation.

Drink plenty of fluids

Fiber acts as a sponge in your colon, absorbing water into stool. As you increase the amount of fiber you eat, make sure you also drink plenty of liquid so that you don't become constipated. Each day, drink at least eight 8-ounce glasses of water or other beverages that don't contain caffeine or alcohol.

Respond to bowel urges

When you need to pass stool, don't delay a trip to the bathroom. Delaying a bowel movement leads to harder stools that require more force to pass, increasing pressure within your colon.

Exercise regularly

Exercise promotes normal bowel function and reduces pressure inside your colon. Try to exercise for 30 to 60 minutes most days of the week. See Chapter 2 for information on what types of exercise to consider.

When you may need medication or surgery

Inflammation or infection in a digestive pouch generally requires more than self-care. Depending on the severity of your symptoms, you may be hospitalized or treated at home. About half the people with diverticulitis, including those with vomiting, fever, high white blood cell count, possible bowel obstruction, or people who are at risk of peritonitis, require hospitalization. You're also more likely to be hospitalized if you are older, are taking steroids, have another disease or have a weakened immune system.

Here are nonsurgical treatments for diverticulitis.

Rest and a restricted diet. A few days of rest allow the infection time to heal. A liquid diet or a diet restricted to low-fiber foods reduces contractions in the colon so that it can rest and heal. In case of severe nausea and vomiting, you may have to avoid all food and take fluids intravenously.

Once your symptoms improve — often in two to four days — you can begin eating more foods, gradually building up to a high-fiber diet.

Antibiotics. Antibiotics kill the bacteria causing the infection. It's important to take the full course of an antibiotic, even if you feel better after a few days.

Painkillers. If your symptoms are accompanied by moderate to severe pain, your doctor may recommend an over-the-counter or prescription analgesic for a few days until the pain improves.

These practices — rest, a low-fiber diet, antibiotics and possibly a painkiller — are often effective for a first attack of diverticulitis. Unfortunately, recurrent episodes are less likely to respond to these simple measures and may require more advanced care.

Your likelihood of having more than one episode of diverticulitis varies. For most people, the risk of recurrence is about 30 percent. You can help prevent a second attack by eating more fiber, drinking plenty of liquids and getting plenty of exercise.

Surgery for diverticulitis

Complications from diverticulitis may include peritonitis, a blockage in your colon, an abscess or a fistula. If one of these occurs, surgery may be needed to fix the problem.

Peritonitis requires emergency surgery, and often a temporary colostomy is required that includes a bag worn outside the body to collect stool. Other problems, such as a narrowing or stricture of the colon, or a fistula, may require an operation after inflammation has subsided, usually about six to eight weeks after the attack. A fistula is an abnormal passageway between two organs, such as the colon and the bladder, resulting from disease in one of the organs.

An abscess can often be drained at the time of the attack. However, surgery may still be needed six to eight weeks later to prevent a recurrence.

To prevent future infections, doctors often recommend that people with recurring diverticulitis have surgery to remove the diseased portion of the colon. There are two forms of surgery.

Primary bowel resection. This is the standard operation for people with diverticulitis who don't need emergency surgery. After the diseased segment of bowel is removed, the colon is rejoined (anastomosis). This maintains the passageway for stool so that your colon can function normally.

The extent of inflammation and other complicating factors, such as obesity, will help determine whether you're a candidate for traditional or laparoscopic surgery. With traditional open surgery, a surgeon makes one long incision in your abdomen. With laparoscopic surgery, three or four small incisions are made in your abdomen. Laparoscopic surgery requires less recovery time. However, laparoscopic surgery isn't generally possible for people who are obese or who have extensive inflammation or infection.

Bowel resection with colostomy. This form of surgery may be necessary if you have extensive inflammation in your colon that makes it unsafe to rejoin your colon and rectum. During the operation, called Hartmann's procedure, a surgeon removes the diseased section of colon, closes off the upper part of the rectum and makes an opening in your abdominal wall. The colon is brought up through this opening and sutured to the abdominal wall to create the colostomy. Stool passes through the colon and into a bag attached to the abdominal wall.

A colostomy may be temporary or permanent. Several months later — once the inflammation has healed — you may consider a second operation to restore continuity between the colon and rectum. It's important that you discuss with your doctor the benefits and risks of such an operation.

Are you at higher risk of cancer?

There's no evidence that diverticulosis or diverticulitis increases your risk of colon or rectal cancer, or the formation of precancerous growths (polyps) in the lining of the colon or rectum. However, diverticular disease can make cancer more difficult to diagnose.

After an episode of diverticulitis, your doctor may suggest a colonoscopy or another screening test to make sure that you don't have cancer of the colon or rectum.

Chapter 11

Gallstones

It's bedtime, but you can't sleep. You feel a continuous pain in your upper abdomen and nothing relieves it — not antacids or pain relievers. You try changing your position. You stand up, bend over, lie down, but nothing helps. After a while you feel nauseated, and the pain seems to spread to your lower chest and back. Finally, you decide to go to the emergency room, worried that you may be having a heart attack.

Key signs and symptoms

- Upper abdominal pain
- Pain in back, chest or right shoulder blade
- Nausea and vomiting

Following an examination and some tests, you find out that it's not your heart but your gallbladder. Gallbladder pain, commonly called a gallbladder attack, occurs when stones in your gallbladder become lodged in the neck of the gallbladder or the cystic duct and obstruct the gallbladder's opening. This leads to a buildup of pressure in the gallbladder, causing constant pain and often nausea.

Gallstones are common. One in 10 Americans has them. In most people they cause no symptoms and require no treatment. But in about 20 percent of people with gallstones, the stones lead to a gallbladder attack. Gallbladder attacks account for one of the most common operations in the United States — gallbladder removal (cholecystectomy). More than 700,000 Americans have their gallbladders removed each year.

How gallstones form

Your gallbladder is a pear-shaped sac 3 to 6 inches long and 1 to 2 inches across at its widest point. It lies under the liver, in the right side of your upper abdomen. The gallbladder stores a digestive fluid called bile, produced in your liver. Bile is composed, in part, of water, electrolytes, cholesterol and bilirubin (bil-ih-ROO-bin). Bilirubin is a greenish yellow waste product excreted by the liver that gives bile its color. If it backs up into your blood, it can cause your skin and eyes to turn yellow (jaundice). Bile also contains bile salts and the chemical lecithin (LES-ih-thin) that together dissolve cholesterol and allow it to be excreted by the liver.

When you eat a meal containing fat or protein, your gallbladder contracts and empties bile through small tubes called bile ducts, which lead to the upper portion of your small intestine (duodenum). The bile helps your small intestine digest and absorb fat and certain vitamins. When bile becomes chemically imbalanced, it can form into hardened particles, which can grow into stones as small as a grain of sand or bigger than a golf ball. Some people have just one stone, while others have multiple stones that may number in the hundreds or even thousands, sometimes referred to as gravel or sand.

Multiple factors contribute to the formation of gallstones, many of which aren't well understood. Factors that are recognized as causing gallstones include the following.

Too much cholesterol. Normally, bile contains enough bile salts and lecithin to dissolve cholesterol that's excreted. But cholesterol isn't easily soluble. If bile has more cholesterol than can be dissolved, the excessive cholesterol can form into crystals and fuse into one or more stones of varying shapes and sizes. Obesity and a genetic predisposition may contribute to this process.

Incomplete or infrequent gallbladder emptying. Your gallbladder may fail to contract and empty as it should. This may occur during pregnancy or prolonged fasting. The longer bile stays in your gallbladder, the more water your gallbladder absorbs and the more concentrated the bile becomes. Bile that's too concentrated can become sludgy and form stones.

Three types

Not all gallstones have the same composition. You may have one of three varieties.

Cholesterol stones. They're made from cholesterol that bile is unable to keep dissolved. About 80 percent of gallstones in people in the United States and Europe are composed predominantly of cholesterol. Some of this type of stone are almost pure cholesterol, but more often these stones also contain considerable amounts of other components, such as bilirubin and calcium. These are sometimes called mixed stones.

Pigment stones. This type of stone forms when bile contains too much bilirubin. Pigment stones are very dark brown or black and generally small. What causes them to form isn't always apparent. Some are associated with excess production of bilirubin stemming from severe scarring of the liver (cirrhosis), or excessive red blood cell destruction and removal (hemolytic anemia).

Primary bile duct stones. Cholesterol and pigment stones that escape and lodge in the bile ducts are known as secondary or retained duct stones. Primary bile duct stones are different in that they actually form within the bile ducts. These stones are usually soft and brown and are made of decomposed bile.

The makings of an attack

Gallstones usually settle at the bottom of your gallbladder, and most of the time they don't cause any problems. Some people associate gallstones with signs and symptoms such as heartburn, indigestion or bloating. However, there's no evidence that gallbladder disease causes these symptoms.

It's when the stones migrate up to the neck (outlet) of the gallbladder that serious problems can occur. When your gallbladder contracts to expel bile into your small intestine, the stones may escape, or try to. Tiny stones usually pass through your bile ducts, enter the small intestine and leave your body without causing problems. But larger stones can get stuck at the entrance to the cystic duct, within a bile duct or at the entrance to the small intestine.

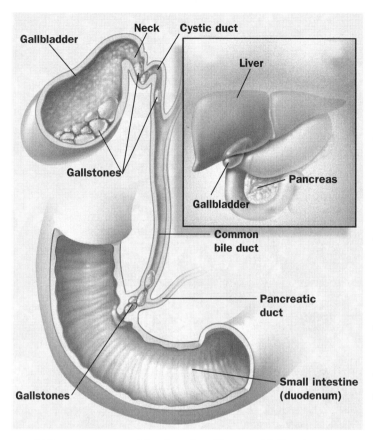

Neck Cystic duct

Gallbladder

Gallstones

Liver

Pancreas

Gallbladder

Common bile duct

Pancreatic duct

Gallstones

Small intestine (duodenum)

Your gallbladder is behind your liver in the upper-right side of your abdomen. A gallbladder attack occurs when stones that form in the gallbladder lodge in the neck of the gallbladder or the cystic duct leading to the common (main) bile duct. Gallstones that obstruct the common bile duct or pancreatic duct can cause inflammation of the bile ducts (cholangitis) or pancreatitis.

When a stone blocks the flow of bile, it causes nausea and steady pain that may be moderate to severe (gallbladder attack). The attack may last from 15 minutes to several hours. Usually, a stone lodged at the entrance to the cystic duct will drop back down to the bottom of your gallbladder after a gallbladder attack has passed. If the stone doesn't work its way free, inflammation and infection may occur in the gallbladder. Other signs and symptoms may include fever, chills, dark-colored urine, jaundice, and pale-colored stools, depending on where a stone is lodged.

These conditions also may occur:

- If the cystic duct remains blocked, your gallbladder could become infected and even rupture. Rupture is rare, however, occurring in only about 10 percent of people with acute inflammation.
- If a stone is lodged in the common bile duct, blocking flow of bile from the liver, you may get jaundice, as well as fever, chills and a blood infection.

- Gallstones that collect at the entrance to the small intestine can block the pancreatic duct, causing inflammation of the pancreas (pancreatitis).

Are you at risk?

Why gallstones develop in some people and not in others is unclear. These factors appear to put you at increased risk.

Being female. Gallstones are twice as common in women as in men. That may be because the hormone estrogen causes the liver to excrete more cholesterol into bile.

Pregnancy, birth control pills and hormone replacement therapy also increase the level of cholesterol in bile and decrease your gallbladder's ability to completely empty bile. However, you shouldn't stop taking birth control pills or hormone replacement therapy simply because you're concerned about gallstones. Talk with your doctor first. The benefits of birth control pills and hormone replacement therapy may outweigh the increased risk of gallstones.

Excess weight. Several studies show that the more you weigh, the greater is your risk. Obese people have a threefold to sevenfold greater risk of developing gallstones than do people whose weight is healthy. People who are overweight tend to accumulate excess cholesterol in their bile. Excess weight also decreases bile salt formation, as well as the ability of your gallbladder to contract and empty.

Diet and dieting. A diet high in fat and sugar, combined with a sedentary lifestyle, increases your risk of gallstones. Fasting and rapid weight-loss diets also increase your risk of gallstone formation by altering levels of bile salts and cholesterol and throwing bile chemistry out of balance.

Some doctors prescribe a bile salt medication (ursodiol) for people in weight-loss programs to offset potential buildup of stone-forming cholesterol. It helps dissolve cholesterol by improving the chemical balance in bile.

Age. Risk of gallstones increases with age. By age 70, about 35 percent of women and 20 percent of men have gallstones. One reason might be that as you get older your body tends to secrete more cholesterol into bile.

Family history. Gallstones often run in families, pointing to a possible genetic link. Two genes that cause gallstones have been identified in mice and are being investigated in humans.

Ethnic group. American Indians have the highest incidence of gallstones in the United States, followed by people of Hispanic origin. Among Pima Indians of Arizona, more than 70 percent of women have gallstones by age 30, and most American Indian men eventually have them. People of Asian or African descent are among the least likely to have gallstones.

Can you prevent gallstones?

Some home remedies recommend that you drink olive oil, apple juice or lemon juice to stimulate the gallbladder to empty out small stones. These practices have no beneficial effect.

The fact is that no diet has been shown to prevent gallstones. But there are two steps you can take to lower your risk. One is to maintain a healthy weight and the other is to avoid crash diets with low intake of calories and rapid weight loss.

Although not scientifically proved, there's some indication that exercise may help prevent gallstones. One study found that men who exercised regularly and vigorously for 30 minutes each day were 34 percent less likely to have gallstone attacks than were men who didn't exercise. Researchers speculate that exercise may help stabilize the chemical balance of bile, inhibiting stone development.

Identifying the stones

If your doctor suspects you have gallstones, you'll probably undergo one or more of the following tests to locate the stones.

Computerized tomography (CT) scan. A CT scan of the abdomen can sometimes reveal gallstones that contain high levels of calcium. In addition, during a gallbladder attack, your gallbladder may appear thickened on a CT or ultrasound scan.

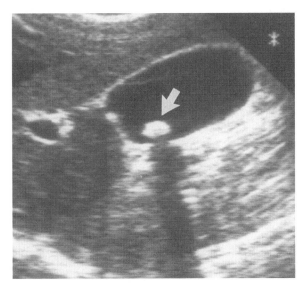

Ultrasound image of a large gallstone (arrow) inside the gallbladder

Ultrasound. This is a painless procedure that lasts only about 15 minutes. Ultrasound can detect stones in your gallbladder with about 95 percent accuracy (see image above). It's much less accurate in detecting stones that have passed into bile ducts.

Radionuclide scan. A small amount of a radioactive tracer material is given intravenously, followed by a scan of the gallbladder to see if the tracer material gains access to the gallbladder. If it doesn't, a stone is likely blocking the opening of the gallbladder or cystic duct.

Blood tests. Elevated levels of certain substances, including bilirubin, alkaline phosphatase and aminotransferases, suggest a bile duct obstruction.

Endoscopic retrograde cholangiopancreatography (ERCP). This procedure allows your doctor to take pictures of your bile ducts. While you're sedated, a flexible tube with an attached camera (endoscope) is threaded through your upper digestive tract to the opening of your common bile duct. Through a catheter located inside the tube, dye is injected into the common bile duct, outlining your bile ducts so that they can be seen on X-ray images. If a stone is discovered in a duct, it usually can be extracted immediately with tools attached to the endoscope.

Treatment options

Usually, the best treatment for gallstones is to do nothing more than watch and wait. This is almost always recommended if you have "silent stones," which typically don't cause any symptoms or other problems. Silent stones often are discovered by accident, during diagnostic testing for another health condition.

If you've had one or more gallbladder attacks, your doctor will probably recommend surgery, unless you have other health problems that make surgery too risky.

Surgery

Surgery to remove the gallbladder, called cholecystectomy (ko-luh-sis-TEK-tuh-me), is generally safe and effective. It's the most common treatment for gallstones because the gallbladder isn't an absolutely essential organ, and new stones usually form if just the stones are removed.

Cholecystectomy is performed one of two ways.

Open surgery. This approach, in which the gallbladder is removed through a large abdominal incision, is used only occasionally today. Your doctor may recommend open surgery if your gallbladder walls are thick and hard, or if you have scar tissue from earlier abdominal operations. Recovery typically involves a week's stay in the hospital, followed by about three weeks at home.

Laparoscopic surgery. The vast majority of gallbladder surgeries are now done by making four small incisions in your abdomen instead of one large one. The surgeon creates room to examine your abdomen by filling it with carbon dioxide. The gas is injected by means of a tube that's inserted through an incision a half-inch to an inch long, near your navel. Three other small incisions are made to insert surgical instruments. One instrument contains a scope to view the gallbladder. Another is equipped with a laser or electric cutting device to remove the gallbladder.

Laparoscopic surgery ordinarily requires only an overnight hospital stay. Recovery time also is shorter because the surgeon doesn't cut through abdominal muscles, which take longer to heal. Other advantages include less postoperative pain and less scarring.

Nonsurgical options

Your doctor may recommend one of these treatments if you have complications or other health problems that make surgery inadvisable. The major disadvantage of these nonsurgical alternatives is that gallstones usually redevelop.

Bile acid dissolution therapy. Bile acid tablets dissolve cholesterol stones over several months or years. However, they don't work on pigment stones. Ursodiol (Actigall) is widely used because it's effective and seems to have the fewest side effects, including mainly occasional, mild diarrhea. Ursodiol works only on stones containing large amounts of cholesterol and no detectable calcium, and when the cystic duct leading to the gallbladder is open, allowing bile to enter and exit normally.

The disadvantage of ursodiol is that its effects aren't permanent. Gallstones tend to recur in about half of people taking ursodiol within five years after treatment, unless the medication is continued indefinitely.

Sound wave therapy. Also known as extracorporeal shock wave lithotripsy, this treatment is more effective and more commonly used for kidney stones than for gallstones. It sends high-frequency sound waves through your abdominal wall to break up gallstones. You then take ursodiol tablets to dissolve the stone fragments. Shock wave therapy works best on single stones less than a half-inch in diameter. Like other treatments in which the gallbladder is left in place, the stone recurrence rate is high without long-term ursodiol treatment.

Life without a gallbladder

Most people who have surgery to remove their gallbladders get along well without them. The liver continues to make enough bile to digest fat in a healthy diet. But instead of being stored in your gallbladder, bile flows out of the liver and empties directly into the small intestine.

You don't need to change your eating habits after surgery. However, with bile flowing more frequently into your small intestine, you may experience a greater number of bowel movements and your stools may be softer. Many times, though, these changes are only temporary. Over time, your intestines usually adjust to the effects of gallbladder removal.

Chapter 12

Pancreatitis

I t's a stomachache such as you've never had before. Pain in your upper abdomen that seems to bore right through to your back. Lying flat causes your stomach to hurt even more, so to relieve the pain, you double over. Pain like this, which may last for hours to days, is typical of pancreatitis (pan-kre-uh-TI-tis), an inflammation of the pancreas.

Key signs and symptoms

- Abdominal pain
- Nausea and vomiting
- Fever
- Bloating and gas
- Foul-smelling, loose, oily stools
- Weight loss

The pancreas is a long, flat gland that lies horizontally behind your stomach. The head of the pancreas rests against the upper part of the small intestine (duodenum), and its tail reaches toward your spleen.

The pancreas has two main functions.

- It produces digestive juices and enzymes that help break down fats, carbohydrates and proteins (pancreatic exocrine function). The juices and enzymes are transported through a small duct that opens into the duodenum.
- It secretes the hormones insulin and glucagon into the bloodstream, along with somatostatin, another hormone that helps regulate their function. The primary role of insulin and glucagon is to regulate the metabolism of carbohydrates.

When inflammation develops in the pancreas, these functions are disrupted. The inflammation can be acute or chronic. Most cases are mild to moderate, but in about 20 percent of people, symptoms can be severe.

Acute vs. chronic

Each year, about 80,000 cases of acute pancreatitis are diagnosed. Acute pancreatitis comes on suddenly. The main symptom is mild to severe pain in your upper abdomen that often radiates to your back and chest. It can persist for hours or days without relief. Drinking alcohol or eating may worsen the pain. Many people with acute pancreatitis sit up and bend forward, or curl up in a fetal position, because these positions seem to relieve the pain. The pain may be so severe that hospitalization is necessary.

Normally, digestive enzymes produced in the pancreas are in an inactive form. It's only when they're transported through the pancreatic ductal system and into the duodenum that these enzymes are activated. However, in acute pancreatitis, these digestive enzymes become activated while still in the pancreas, causing irritation, inflammation and sometimes destruction of delicate pancreatic tissues.

People with severe inflammation often feel and look very sick, and they frequently experience nausea and vomiting. Other symptoms may include a high fever, difficulty breathing and abdominal bruises from internal bleeding.

Chronic pancreatitis differs from acute pancreatitis in that the inflammation happens over time, often many years. In the early stages of chronic pancreatitis, you may experience mild to severe episodes similar to acute pancreatitis. However, because damage to the pancreas occurs more slowly, chronic pancreatitis may be more difficult to diagnose than acute pancreatitis.

While a few people with chronic pancreatitis have no pain, most have intermittent periods of mild to moderate abdominal pain. The pain may be sharp and last for a few hours, or it may be a continuous dull ache that lasts for weeks. In addition to pain, you may experience nausea and vomiting, fever, bloating and gas. Drinking alcohol or eating can make symptoms worse.

Unlike acute pancreatitis, which often resolves spontaneously without long-term complications, chronic disease usually causes permanent damage. As the inflammation persists, it slowly destroys tissues in the pancreas. The organ is less able to secrete the enzymes and hormones needed for proper digestion. This leads to malabsorption of nutrients, particularly fat, causing weight loss and passage of fat-containing stools that are loose, foul-smelling and oily in appearance. Eventually, the cells that produce insulin are impaired, causing diabetes. Unfortunately, warnings of malabsorption and diabetes often don't appear until much of the gland has been destroyed.

Two causes stand out

Pancreatitis can occur for various reasons, and in some cases its cause is unknown. The two most common known causes are excessive alcohol use and gallstones.

Alcohol

Heavy alcohol use over many years is a leading cause of chronic pancreatitis. Excessive alcohol may also cause an acute attack. Up to 70 percent of cases of chronic pancreatitis and about 35 percent of cases of acute pancreatitis in the United States are linked to consumption of excessive amounts of alcohol.

It's unclear how alcohol damages the pancreas. One theory is that excessive alcohol leads to protein plugs — precursors to small stones — that form in the pancreas and block parts of the pancreatic duct. Another theory is that alcohol directly injures pancreatic tissues.

Gallstones

About half the people with acute pancreatitis have gallstones. Sometimes these stones will migrate out of the gallbladder through the common bile duct, which merges with the pancreatic duct near the entrance to the duodenum. At this junction, gallstones can lodge in or near the pancreatic duct and block the flow of pancreatic juices into the duodenum. Digestive enzymes activate in the pancreas instead of the digestive tract, causing acute pancreatitis.

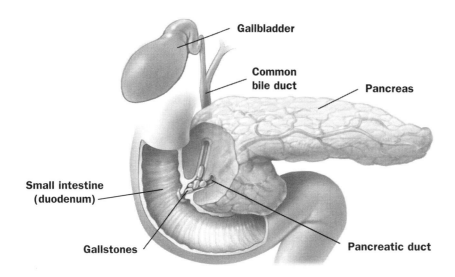

Gallbladder

Common
bile duct

Pancreas

Small intestine
(duodenum)

Gallstones

Pancreatic duct

Gallstones that leave the gallbladder and block the pancreatic duct are a common cause of acute pancreatitis. Digestive juices produced by the pancreas are trapped there, inflaming delicate tissues.

Less common causes

Other conditions that may lead to acute pancreatitis include:

- Calcium deposits or stones that can block the pancreatic or common bile duct
- Increased levels of triglycerides (blood fats) or of calcium in blood (hypercalcemia)
- Structural abnormalities of the pancreas, abdominal trauma or major surgery
- A bacterial or viral infection
- Inherited genetic mutations, most notably in the cationic trypsinogen gene

Occasionally, a complication of acute pancreatitis can lead to chronic pancreatitis. Sometimes, young adults with cystic fibrosis and associated gene abnormalities have episodes of chronic pancreatitis. Some people also are born with a hereditary form of the disease that can cause attacks during childhood or adolescence.

In approximately 20 percent of people with chronic pancreatitis, and 10 percent of people with acute disease, no cause is apparent. However, researchers suspect some acute attacks may be linked to gallstones that are too small to identify. Others may involve unidentified genetic mutations.

Treating acute pancreatitis

If your doctor suspects acute pancreatitis, he or she will check your abdomen for pain and tenderness. A sample of your blood also may be analyzed for abnormalities that can signal acute inflammation, such as:

- Elevated levels of the pancreatic enzymes amylase and lipase
- An elevated white blood cell count
- Elevated levels of liver enzymes and bilirubin, a substance that results from the breakdown of red blood cells
- High blood sugar (hyperglycemia)
- A low calcium level (High calcium levels can cause pancreatitis, but low levels of calcium in blood, called hypocalcemia, are a result of acute pancreatitis.)

Your doctor may request an ultrasound or computerized tomography (CT) scan of your abdomen to examine the pancreas and look for gallstones, a duct problem or destruction of the gland. You also may have X-rays of your abdomen and chest to rule out other causes of your pain.

Treatment of severe acute pancreatitis usually requires a hospital stay. If you have complications, you may be admitted to the intensive care unit. Treatment focuses on controlling pain, aggressive hydration, and identifying and treating complications. Resting the pancreas by avoiding eating also may be done. Feeding through a tube that's threaded through the nose, down the esophagus and past the stomach into the small intestine may help resolve pancreatic inflammation and possibly prevent infection.

If your attack is caused by gallstones blocking the pancreatic duct, your doctor may recommend a procedure to remove the stones. You may eventually need surgery to remove the gallbladder if gallstones continue to pose problems. If alcohol is the cause, treatment may include therapy to stop drinking. However, complete abstinence from alcohol doesn't guarantee you won't have another attack.

Mild cases of acute pancreatitis generally improve in three to seven days, after which you may be able to eat and drink again. Moderate to severe cases may take longer.

Complications of acute pancreatitis

Acute pancreatitis may lead to destruction (necrosis) of part of the pancreas, inflammation and fluid buildup in and around the gland, and failure of other organs, including the heart, lungs and kidneys. Between 15 percent and 30 percent of all cases of acute pancreatitis are severe and may lead to complications.

Infection. A damaged pancreas may become infected with bacteria that spread from the small intestine into the pancreas. Signs of infection include fever, an elevated white blood cell count and organ failure. A fluid sample from the pancreas may be tested for bacterial infection. If the tests are positive, you'll receive antibiotics. Some people also need surgery to drain or remove infected areas of the pancreas. Sometimes, multiple operations are necessary.

Pseudocysts. Cyst-like blisters called pseudocysts may form on and extend from the pancreas after an attack of acute pancreatitis. If the cyst is small, no special treatment is necessary. If it is large, becomes infected or causes bleeding, intervention is necessary. Your doctor may drain the cyst through a catheter or you may need surgery to remove the cyst.

Abscess. This is a collection of pus near the pancreas that can develop three to four weeks after the onset of acute pancreatitis. Treatment involves drainage of the abscess by catheter or surgery.

Treating chronic pancreatitis

To confirm a diagnosis of chronic pancreatitis, your doctor will likely take samples of your blood and your stool. Blood tests can identify abnormalities associated with chronic pancreatitis and help rule out acute inflammation. The stool test is to measure the fat content in your feces. Chronic pancreatitis often causes excess fat in your stool because the fat isn't digested and absorbed in your small intestine.

Your doctor may have you undergo X-ray, ultrasound or endoscopic procedures to look for evidence of a blockage in the pancreatic duct or common bile duct. If you've lost weight or your doctor suspects a malabsorption problem, you may receive a stimulation test. A solution is injected in your bloodstream to stimulate the pancreas. The gland's ability to discharge secretions into the duodenum is then measured. You may also need additional tests if your doctor is concerned about the possibility of other diseases, such as pancreatic cancer. Having chronic pancreatitis puts you at a slightly higher risk of pancreatic cancer.

The main goals of treatment for chronic pancreatitis are to control pain and treat malabsorption problems.

Relieving pain

Unlike acute pancreatitis, in which the pain often disappears within a few days to weeks, with chronic pancreatitis the pain can linger. Persistent pain can be the biggest challenge of chronic pancreatitis. In addition to conventional pain relievers, your doctor may prescribe pancreatic enzymes. Enzyme therapy works by increasing the levels of enzymes in the duodenum, which in turn decreases the secretion of enzymes by the pancreas. This is thought to reduce secretion pressure — and hence, pain — within the pancreas.

For severe pain that can't be controlled, treatment options include surgery to remove damaged tissue or procedures to block pain signals or deaden those nerves transmitting the pain.

Enzyme therapy for malabsorption

Enzyme supplements taken with each meal, such as pancrelipase (Pancrease, Viokase), can treat malabsorption problems caused by the pancreas. The tablets replace those digestive enzymes that are not secreted by the pancreas, helping to restore normal digestion. Depending on the preparation, you may take up to eight tablets with meals — two tablets after eating a few bites, four during the meal, and two after the meal. You may also need to take the tablets with snacks.

Treating diabetes

Chronic pancreatitis can cause diabetes. Treatment is similar to that of type 2 diabetes (formerly called adult-onset or noninsulin-dependent diabetes) and usually involves maintaining a healthy diet and getting regular exercise. Some people also need insulin injections. Your doctor can explain how to manage your diabetes, recognize symptoms of high and low blood sugar, and prevent complications.

Managing pancreatitis

People with chronic pancreatitis often have lifelong signs and symptoms, such as pain and malabsorption of certain nutrients. Most people with acute pancreatitis, on the other hand, recover completely. But even if you experience no lingering symptoms, it's still important to try to keep your pancreas as healthy as possible.

Avoid alcohol. If you can't voluntarily stop drinking alcohol, get treatment for alcoholism. Abstaining from alcohol may not reduce your pain, but it will reduce your risk of dying of your disease.

Stop smoking. Smoking has several bad effects for people with pancreatitis. It reduces pancreatic function, hastens the development of stones and increases the risk of pancreatic cancer.

Eat smaller meals. The more you eat during a meal, the greater the amount of digestive juices your pancreas must produce. Instead of large meals, eat smaller, more frequent meals.

Limit fat in your diet. This will help reduce loose and oily stools that result when your small intestine isn't able to absorb fat. Discuss with your doctor or a dietitian how much fat to eat each day to prevent complications from too little fat in your diet.

Follow a diet high in carbohydrates. Carbohydrates give you energy to help fight fatigue. They're found in foods made from starches (complex carbohydrates) or sugars (simple carbohydrates). At least 55 percent to 65 percent of your daily calories should come from carbohydrates. Try to get most of these calories from complex carbohydrates found in grains, vegetables and legumes.

Find safe ways to control pain. Talk with your doctor about options for controlling your pain, including the benefits and risks of prescription and over-the-counter pain relievers. Although often effective, these medications do carry side effects, including dependence and stomach problems.

Chapter 13

Liver disease

People don't often associate digestive problems with the liver. But lack of appetite, weight loss and nausea may stem from a liver disorder rather than a stomach or intestinal problem. There are more than 100 liver diseases and conditions.

The liver is a complex organ with many functions. One function is to process (metabolize) nutrients absorbed by your small intestine and convert them into forms your body can use. Another function of the liver is to filter waste and toxins from your blood. If your liver isn't working properly, your body may not be getting the nutrients it needs, leading to weight loss and fatigue. Buildup of waste and toxins in your blood can cause yellowing of your skin and eyes (jaundice), loss of appetite, nausea and, sometimes, vomiting.

Hepatitis

The most common liver disease is hepatitis, inflammation of the liver. There are several forms of hepatitis.

Alcohol- or drug-induced hepatitis. This is the most common form of hepatitis, occurring in people who drink excessive amounts of alcohol or take certain medications. The inflammation stems from toxic chemicals that your body produces as it breaks down alcohol and drugs. Over time, these chemicals can damage liver cells and interfere with your liver's ability to do its job.

Up to 35 percent of heavy drink-
ers get alcoholic hepatitis, although
the condition may often go undiagnosed. Women develop alcoholic
hepatitis after a shorter period and
with smaller amounts of alcohol
abuse than do men.

Medications that most commonly
lead to drug-induced hepatitis are
nonprescription pain relievers,
especially if the drugs are taken

> **Key signs and symptoms**
>
> - Fatigue
> - Loss of appetite
> - Nausea
> - Unexplained weight loss
> - Yellowing of skin and eyes (jaundice)

frequently or combined with alcohol. Nonprescription pain relievers include acetaminophen (Tylenol, others) and nonsteroidal anti-
inflammatory drugs (NSAIDs), such as aspirin, ibuprofen (Advil,
Motrin, others), naproxen (Aleve) and ketoprofen (Orudis).

Prescription medications also can lead to liver difficulties, including hepatitis. In most people, the following drugs don't cause
any problems. But in some people with liver disease or other health
problems, these drugs can be damaging:

- Valproic acid, an antiseizure medication
- Methotrexate, a cancer medication also used to treat psoriasis
  and rheumatoid arthritis
- The statin family of cholesterol medications, including
  atorvastatin, lovastatin, pravastatin and simvastatin
- Certain high blood pressure medications, including calcium
  channel blockers and angiotensin-converting enzyme (ACE)
  inhibitors
- Certain antibiotics
- Some diabetes medications

Hepatitis A. This highly contagious form of hepatitis is spread
by food or water that's contaminated by the feces of someone who
has hepatitis A. It's estimated that about one in three Americans
has evidence of past infection. Outbreaks of hepatitis A in the
United States have been traced to strawberries, green onions and
other produce that may have been contaminated by irrigation
water or by an infected worker who failed to wash his or her hands

properly before handling the food. Hepatitis A is the form of hepatitis you're most likely to encounter during international travel. It usually resolves itself without treatment. In a few cases, especially in older adults, hepatitis A may cause severe symptoms requiring medical treatment and perhaps hospitalization. In rare cases, it can be fatal.

Hepatitis B. This virus also is highly contagious. It's found in blood, semen and saliva and can survive for seven days or more outside the body. It's commonly transmitted through unprotected sexual contact and by sharing contaminated syringes and needles during intravenous drug use. People at greatest risk of the disease are those with multiple sexual partners, users of illicit drugs and hospital workers who are exposed to blood and blood products. More than 1.25 million Americans have hepatitis B. Each year 78,000 new cases are diagnosed. Worldwide, about 300 million people are carriers of the hepatitis B virus. Infection is more common in men than in women.

Hepatitis C. Hepatitis C is the most common cause of viral hepatitis in the United States. It's spread through blood and blood products and contaminated needles. Users of illicit intravenous or intranasal drugs who share paraphernalia account for about 38 percent of new infections. People who received blood transfusions before 1992 also are at increased risk of hepatitis C. In 1992, blood banks began screening for the virus. Because this form of hepatitis can take decades to progress, it's unclear how many of the people who had blood transfusions before 1992 may be infected. Contrary to popular myth, hepatitis C isn't spread through breast-feeding, hugging, sneezing, coughing, consuming food or water that contains the virus, or sharing eating and drinking utensils.

In the United States alone, more than 2.7 million people are chronically infected with hepatitis C. About 20 percent to 30 percent of people with the virus develop scarring (cirrhosis) of the liver. Hepatitis C is also the leading reason for liver transplants. Each year, 8,000 to 10,000 people die of liver failure stemming from hepatitis C. The Centers for Disease Control and Prevention estimates that illness and death due to hepatitis C infection will increase two to three times in the next 10 to 20 years.

Screening for hepatitis C

A simple screening test can pinpoint hepatitis C antibodies in blood, often identifying the disease before symptoms develop and serious liver damage occurs. Have a screening test if you:

- Are using or have used illicit intravenous or intranasal drugs (even once)
- Received a blood transfusion before 1992
- Received a transplanted organ before 1992
- Received blood-clotting factor before 1987
- Have been accidentally exposed to the blood of others
- Are undergoing hemodialysis (or have undergone in the past)
- Have hemophilia
- Have had sexual relations or have shared razors, toothbrushes or nail clippers with someone who has hepatitis C

Hepatitis D. To get this blood-borne virus you must already have had hepatitis B. Hepatitis D survives and replicates by attaching itself to the hepatitis B virus. Hepatitis D is not common in the United States and is most prevalent among people people with hemophilia and people with diabetes who must regularly use a needle stick to check their blood sugar level.

Hepatitis E. A food-borne virus similar to hepatitis A, this virus is prevalent in Asia and South America. Most cases of hepatitis E reported in the United States involve travelers to parts of the world where the virus is common.

Autoimmune hepatitis. This form of hepatitis is more common among women than men, typically occurring between ages 15 and 40. The disease is believed to result from a trigger that causes the immune system to attack liver cells. Suspected triggers include the measles virus, the Epstein-Barr virus which causes mononucleosis, and viral forms of hepatitis.

Nonalcoholic fatty liver disease (NAFLD). In this condition — sometimes also referred to as nonalcoholic steatohepatitis — the liver contains excessive fat deposits, similar to alcohol-induced hepatitis. But the condition is not caused by alcohol abuse.

NAFLD most often occurs in people who are obese or who have diabetes or high cholesterol levels. It also may occur in people who take steroids or who are malnourished. NAFLD is increasingly recognized as a common cause of abnormalities seen in liver test results.

Acute versus chronic hepatitis

Hepatitis symptoms may last for a short period and then disappear (acute hepatitis), or they may last for a lifetime (chronic hepatitis).

Acute hepatitis. Acute hepatitis generally causes little or no permanent liver damage. It may develop suddenly or gradually, but it usually subsides in six months or less. As your body's defenses overcome the virus, liver inflammation and associated signs and symptoms subside and then disappear. Hepatitis A and E are acute forms. Hepatitis B also is acute, but in a few cases the inflammation can become chronic. Infants born with hepatitis B usually have chronic disease.

Chronic hepatitis. In this condition, the liver remains inflamed, even though you may not have any symptoms. Some people have hepatitis for more than 20 years without realizing it. Over time, the inflammation can cause scar tissue to form in the liver (cirrhosis), eventually leading to liver failure. People with cirrhosis also are at increased risk of liver cancer.

Most forms of hepatitis C are chronic. Hepatitis C may begin as an acute infection, but the disease often becomes chronic. Hepatitis C accounts for between 60 percent and 70 percent of all chronic cases of viral hepatitis. It's considered a major health threat because people who have the disease for years without knowing it may pass it on to others. Chronic hepatitis can take different routes. It may progress very slowly and damage only a limited portion of the liver, or it may progress rapidly, causing extensive liver damage.

Diagnosing hepatitis

Because hepatitis often differs from one person to another, there aren't any common warning signs of the disease. If your doctor suspects your symptoms may be related to hepatitis, he or she will begin by asking you questions about your health and lifestyle. Did you have a blood transfusion before 1992? Have you recently visited a foreign country? Do you practice unsafe sex or use self-injected illicit drugs?

A physical examination is generally the next step. Your doctor will feel (palpate) your upper abdomen for an enlarged, shrunken or hardened liver. He or she will also look for other warning signs of liver disease — swelling of the abdomen, legs, and ankles, and yellowing of the skin and eyes (jaundice). In addition to an exam, you'll take blood tests. In people who don't have symptoms, a routine blood donation or a blood test for another condition is often the way the disease is first detected.

Blood tests for liver disease, called liver tests or liver function tests, can identify four types of abnormalities.

Liver cell damage. If liver cells are inflamed or damaged, enzymes normally found in those cells will leak into the bloodstream. Two tests that check for elevated enzyme levels are the alanine aminotransferase and aspartate aminotransferase tests.

Reduced liver function. When your liver is impaired, usually because of severe liver injury, it isn't able to produce the amount of protein (albumin) it normally does, or provide certain blood-clotting factors (prothrombin). Albumin level and prothrombin time (PT) tests measure these functions.

Increased levels of liver alkaline phosphatase. This enzyme is produced by cells located in bile ducts in your liver. The levels may increase with conditions that affect the bile ducts.

Increased bilirubin. Bilirubin is a substance that results from breakdown of red blood cells. If your liver isn't removing bilirubin normally, elevated levels circulate in your bloodstream. This test is simply called a bilirubin test.

Blood tests often provide sufficient information to make a diagnosis of hepatitis. However, your doctor may want to remove (biopsy) and examine liver tissue samples. These biopsy specimens can help identify the specific type of hepatitis you have. They also indicate the severity of the inflammation and the extent of any permanent liver damage.

Treating hepatitis

Treatment depends on the type of hepatitis. If you have hepatitis A, you probably won't need any medication. However, you may require hospitalization if you're pregnant, older, dehydrated, or you have other health problems. In rare cases when hepatitis A leads to liver failure, a liver transplant may be considered.

Treatment for other forms of hepatitis is still evolving. The primary goals of medical care are to relieve symptoms and prevent scarring (cirrhosis) of the liver. For viral forms of hepatitis, another important goal is to reduce or eliminate the amount of the virus in body fluids (viral levels). Your treatment may include one or more of the following approaches.

Corticosteroids. Steroids reduce liver inflammation by suppressing the immune system. These drugs are used to treat chronic autoimmune hepatitis, causing short-term relief of symptoms (remission) in about 65 percent of people who take them. However, relapse occurs in about 50 percent within six months of withdrawal of medication, and in about 80 percent within three years. Steroids aren't prescribed for viral forms of hepatitis because suppressing the immune system encourages the virus to multiply more rapidly.

The two most commonly used steroids are prednisone and prednisolone. Side effects of these medications include weight gain, skin problems, elevated blood pressure, diabetes, cataracts, infection, osteoporosis and a moon-shaped face. Once your disease is in remission, your doctor may gradually reduce the dosage to the lowest possible level to avoid or lessen the side effects.

Interferons. Interferons are a group of naturally occurring compounds that inhibit viruses from replicating. People with hepatitis B or C aren't able to produce enough interferons to ward off the hepatitis virus. To boost interferon, synthetic forms are injected.

Currently, the treatment that has shown the most promise involves a specially constituted form of interferon (pegylated), which is given by injection once a week along with the drug ribavirin, given in pill form twice a day. The sustained response rate (no virus detected six months or more after stopping therapy) is about 55 percent among those who've never been treated with interferon. However, in nearly all cases the virus eventually recurs and requires additional treatment.

Because of its side effects, interferon isn't recommended for people with a history of major depression, low blood cell counts, autoimmune disease, or who abuse alcohol or drugs. Side effects include flu-like symptoms, fatigue, depression and reduced white blood cell and blood platelet counts. Ribavirin has been associated with anemia.

Lamivudine. This medication also interferes with the ability of the hepatitis B virus to reproduce. Initially, it's often quite effective in reducing liver inflammation and viral levels associated with hepatitis B. But over time, the virus can become resistant to the medication. Originally approved for treatment of AIDS, lamivudine also has been approved by the Food and Drug Administration for treatment of hepatitis B. The drug, taken as a tablet, seems to be well tolerated by most people. The most common side effects are fatigue, headache, and ear, nose and throat infections.

Adefovir. This antiviral drug was first used against the human immunodeficiency virus (HIV), but was found to have unacceptable side effects. However, used in lower doses against hepatitis B, adefovir has been effective, especially when treating lamivudine-resistant strains of the virus.

Liver transplantation. When liver damage is extensive and medications are no longer helpful, your doctor may discuss the possibility of a liver transplant. Hepatitis C now accounts for 30 percent of all liver transplants. If you have hepatitis C or B, there's a chance that the hepatitis virus will recur in your new liver. Liver transplant recipients with hepatitis B routinely receive immunoglobulin injections and medication to reduce the risk of recurrence.

Living with hepatitis

Once you have hepatitis, your risk of getting another form is increased. Therefore, it's important to stay as healthy as possible and avoid exposing yourself to additional hepatitis risks. Because hepatitis has several different causes, self-care varies. But the following lifestyle changes generally apply to all forms.

Rest. If you have acute hepatitis, get adequate rest, drink plenty of fluids and eat a high-calorie diet. This will help strengthen your immune system so that you can fight off the virus.

Avoid alcohol. Alcohol can aggravate inflammation and speed progression of cirrhosis and liver failure.

Use medications carefully. Many medications can impair the liver, especially if taken constantly. In addition, if your liver isn't functioning properly, it may not be able to remove toxic wastes produced by medications. Take only medications, including over-the-counter drugs, that you've discussed with your doctor.

Maintain a healthy lifestyle. This includes eating a healthy diet and getting adequate exercise. In addition to improving your physical health, good nutrition and exercise can help overcome depression, a common condition in people with hepatitis.

Preventing hepatitis

These precautions can help you avoid viral forms of hepatitis.

Immunization. There are effective vaccines for preventing hepatitis A and B. Depending on the type of vaccine used, a series of two or three injections offers about 20 years of hepatitis A protection. A series of three injections protects you for at least 10 years against hepatitis B.

Food preparation. Follow these safe-food-handling habits:

- Always thoroughly wash fruits and vegetables.
- Cook foods thoroughly. Freezing doesn't kill viruses.
- When visiting developing countries, use only bottled water for drinking, cooking and brushing your teeth, or tap water that's been boiled for at least 10 minutes.

Workplace precautions. In health care settings, follow all infection control procedures, including hand washing and wearing gloves. In child-care settings, wash hands thoroughly after changing or handling diapers.

Other precautions. Practice these good health habits:

- Follow safe sexual practices. If you have sexual relations with multiple partners, use a latex condom with each sexual contact.
- Don't share drug syringes.
- If you undergo acupuncture, make sure the needles have been sterilized.
- Avoid body piercing and tattooing.
- Don't share toothbrushes, razors, nail clippers or other items that may come into contact with blood.

Hemochromatosis

Hemochromatosis is a genetic abnormality that causes your intestines to absorb too much iron from your diet, which can lead to iron overload. The extra iron enters your bloodstream and builds up in certain organs, primarily the liver. Left untreated, hemochromatosis can lead to organ damage, diabetes and darkening of your skin (sometimes called bronze diabetes). The good news is that unlike hepatitis, hemochromatosis is easily treated.

Key signs and symptoms

- Fatigue
- Joint pain
- Impotence or loss of sex drive
- Increased skin pigmentation (bronzing)
- Increased thirst and urination

If discovered early, it generally causes no permanent damage.

A gene flaw

In rare cases, iron overload may stem from repeated blood transfusions or overconsumption of dietary iron. But by far the most common cause of the disease is a mutation in the gene — the HFE gene, discovered in 1996 — that controls the amount of iron you absorb from food. Exactly how the genetic defect causes iron overload isn't known. Researchers speculate that it holds the blueprint for a faulty protein that leads your intestines to overabsorb iron.

Researchers estimate that approximately one in 10 whites carries a flawed HFE gene, most commonly Americans of Northern European descent. Gene carriers — people with just one abnormal copy — usually don't have problems with iron overload. It's among people with two copies of the abnormal gene that significant iron overload may develop. About 1 in 200 to 1 in 500 Americans has two abnormal copies, which occur by inheriting an abnormal gene from each parent.

Identifying the problem

A blood test called a transferrin saturation test is generally the first step in diagnosing hemochromatosis. If the test shows that you have too much iron in your blood, your doctor may order additional blood tests to further determine iron amounts and to assess the health of your liver. These may include a genetic test to see if you carry two abnormal copies of the HFE gene. To determine the extent of your disease, your doctor may recommend a liver biopsy.

Many people live with high iron levels for years, and by the time hemochromatosis is diagnosed they already may have some liver damage. This disorder often goes undiagnosed in premenopausal women for a longer time because they lose blood each month through menstruation. Their iron levels decrease, delaying symptoms. The average time from onset of symptoms to diagnosis of hemochromatosis is about 10 years.

Blood-letting to remove iron

Treatment for hemochromatosis involves removing excess iron from your blood. You need to have regular blood draws, called blood-letting, or phlebotomy. Once or twice a week a pint of blood is withdrawn from a vein in your arm, in the same way as you make a blood donation. This continues until your iron level returns to normal.

Should you be screened?

Some experts recommend that all adults have a transferrin saturation test at least once during their lifetime — preferably in early adulthood — to measure the iron level in their blood. Others recommend checking for iron overload if there's a family history of hemochromatosis, or signs and symptoms of the condition. Screening for hemochromatosis isn't usually included in routine blood tests. If you want to be tested, you may have to request it.

Experts don't recommend genetic screening all adults because the test is expensive, and it's unclear how many people with this genetic defect have iron overload. However, if you have a close blood relative with hemochromatosis, such as a brother, sister or parent, you may want to have a genetic test to make sure you aren't at risk. If you do carry two abnormal copies of the HFE gene but complications haven't yet developed from the disease, you and your doctor can take steps to prevent future problems.

Your body normally contains 1.5 to 2 grams of stored iron. People with hemochromatosis can have up to 40 grams. Each blood draw removes only about 250 milligrams of iron, so it may take several months to a few years to remove all of the excess iron. After reaching a normal iron level, most people continue to need blood draws four to eight times a year to keep iron from building up.

If the disease has damaged your liver or other organs, you may also need treatment to prevent further organ damage. This may include medication or surgery.

Reducing iron in your diet

It's not necessary or advisable to remove all iron from your diet, but you want to avoid consuming more than the recommended daily amount, 18 milligrams. Products highest in iron are iron supplements and multivitamins. Your doctor may recommend that you avoid them.

In addition to reducing iron intake, you also want to avoid alcohol and limit excessive consumption of vitamin C. Alcohol aggravates liver disease. Vitamin C facilitates iron absorption. Consuming excessive amounts of vitamin C may increase your iron level.

Other inherited liver diseases

Wilson's disease. In this condition, your body accumulates excessive amounts of copper, leading to organ damage. Like hemochromatosis, Wilson's disease stems from a flawed gene. Nearly everyone with the disease has symptoms by age 40, which may include liver tenderness, weight loss, fatigue, mild jaundice and neurologic problems. If caught early, Wilson's disease is treatable with medications that remove excess copper from your body.

Alpha-1-antitrypsin deficiency. This disorder results from a genetic defect that causes your body to produce abnormal forms of the alpha-1-antitrypsin protein, an enzyme inhibitor. The deficiency may lead to lung and liver disease. Most people with alpha-1-antitrypsin deficiency don't develop serious liver disease.

Gilbert syndrome. This mild disorder doesn't lead to liver damage, but jaundice may develop periodically, as may symptoms resembling those of mild liver disease.

Cirrhosis

Almost any chronic liver disease can lead to cirrhosis, a condition in which scar tissue forms in the liver and keeps it from functioning normally. Most often, cirrhosis is the byproduct of chronic liver inflammation caused by chronic alcohol abuse or chronic hepatitis. Cirrhosis can also result from hemochromatosis, Wilson's disease or alpha-1-antitrypsin deficiency.

Here are some other causes of cirrhosis.

Primary biliary cirrhosis. Tiny bile ducts in the liver inflame and scar for unknown reasons. Primary biliary cirrhosis occurs far more often among women than men, generally between the ages of 30 and 60. Complications of the disease may include inflamed joints, osteoporosis from calcium loss, and sicca syndrome, a condition in which your tear glands and salivary glands fail to produce enough lubrication. Some people with the disease live normal lives and never develop signs and symptoms.

Primary sclerosing cholangitis. In this condition, which may stem from an autoimmune disorder, the walls of bile ducts inside and outside the liver thicken and close. About 70 percent of

> ## Key signs and symptoms
> - Loss of appetite
> - Weight loss
> - Weakness and fatigue
> - Abdominal swelling
> - Yellowing of skin and eyes (jaundice)
> - Gastrointestinal bleeding (varices)
> - Sleepiness or confusion

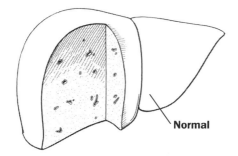 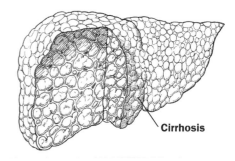

A normal liver (left), shown in cross section, shows no sign of scarring. The cirrhotic liver (right) shows extensive scarring.

people with the disease are men, and many of them also have inflammatory bowel disease.

Identifying cirrhosis

An enlarged, firm liver can signal liver injury. However, as cirrhosis advances, the liver may shrivel. Swelling of your abdomen from accumulation of fluid (ascites) may be another warning sign of the disease. Most often, though, cirrhosis is first suspected after blood tests indicate that your liver isn't functioning properly.

To determine the extent of your disease, your doctor may want to see pictures of your liver by way of ultrasound, computerized tomography (CT) or magnetic resonance imaging (MRI). In addition, you may need a liver biopsy. As with other liver diseases, a biopsy is the only way to definitively diagnose cirrhosis. It may also help determine the cause of liver disease.

Slowing the disease's progression

There is no cure for cirrhosis, and the damage is irreversible. However, the disease often progresses slowly and there are things you can do to reduce further liver damage.

Stop using alcohol. Alcohol breaks down into various chemicals, some of which are toxic to your liver. If you have cirrhosis, avoiding alcohol can increase your survival time.

Limit medications. Because your damaged liver is unable to detoxify and eliminate medications normally from your system, discuss all medications, including nonprescription drugs, with your doctor. Be especially careful not to combine the pain reliever acetaminophen (Tylenol, others) or any other analgesic with alcohol, even if you take only the recommended daily amount of the drug.

Avoid people who are sick. When your liver is damaged, you can't fight off infections as easily as healthy people. Do everything that's reasonable to avoid getting sick. Get vaccinated for hepatitis A and B, influenza and pneumococcal pneumonia.

Eat plenty of fresh fruit, vegetables and whole grains. These foods are high in nutrients, including vitamins A, C and E. Cirrhosis tends to deplete these important vitamins. Your doctor also may prescribe supplemental vitamins K, A and D, because your body may not be getting an adequate amount. However, don't take any supplemental vitamins without your doctor's recommendation.

Restrict salt. The sodium in salt causes some people to retain fluid. So does cirrhosis. Reducing salt may help reduce fluid buildup.

Monitor protein in your diet. Rarely is it necessary to restrict protein in your diet, but it's important that you don't eat excessive amounts. If your cirrhosis is advanced, excessive protein may lead to a condition called hepatic encephalopathy (en-sef-uh-LOP-uh-thee). It's an alteration in your mental condition that occurs when your liver is no longer capable of removing some toxic elements from your blood, such as ammonia, found in proteins. These toxins can affect your brain, causing personality changes, mental confusion, drowsiness or tremors.

Treating complications
Medical treatment for cirrhosis will differ, according to its cause and symptoms. The main focus of medical care often is treating complications.

Liver transplantation for cirrhosis

A liver transplant is generally considered when the disease has advanced to the point when the liver can no longer function. The success rate of liver transplantation continues to improve, and more than 90 percent of people who receive transplants are still alive one year later. The problem is that there are more people in need of liver transplants than there are available donors. In addition, when cirrhosis is related to viral hepatitis, there's a chance the disease will recur in the new liver.

Researchers are studying alternatives to traditional liver transplantation that one day may allow more people to receive lifesaving treatment. In one procedure, a portion of healthy liver (about 60 percent) is removed from a living donor, generally a relative or friend. The failing liver in the person with cirrhosisis is removed and replaced with the healthy liver. Because liver tissue naturally regenerates, the liver should return to normal size and function in two to four weeks in both the donor and the recipient.

Therapies to prevent internal bleeding. Cirrhosis can slow or block blood movement through your liver, causing the formation of small, twisted veins with thin walls. These blood vessels (varices) most commonly occur in the stomach or esophagus. Because the walls of the vessels are subjected to high pressure, it's not uncommon for them to bleed. In an attempt to stop internal bleeding, your doctor may recommend a medication to lower the pressure within the varices or a procedure to prevent blood from flowing into them.

Therapy to reduce fluid retention. Diuretics help reduce accumulation of excess abdominal fluid. To reduce fluid retention, your doctor may ask you to restrict your sodium intake, including cutting down on table salt.

Sometimes, abdominal fluid can become infected, causing pain and fever. If this occurs, your doctor may insert a catheter into your abdomen to remove a fluid sample so that the infecting organism can be identified and the proper antibiotic prescribed.

Medications to reduce itching. Antihistamines as well as cholestyramine (Questran) and rifampin (Rifadin, Rimactane) are prescribed to reduce itching caused by toxins (bile acids) in blood.

Treatments for hepatic encephalopathy. The medication lactulose (Kristalose, Cephulac, others) can help lower blood ammonia levels. Your doctor may recommend an antibiotic to reduce the level of bacteria in your intestines that produce ammonia.

Chapter 14

Cancer

When digestive problems first occur, what people sometimes fear is cancer. Although cancer isn't the cause in most instances, sometimes it is. Signs and symptoms such as bleeding, difficulty swallowing, unexplained weight loss and a change in bowel habits can be warning signs of gastrointestinal cancer. Cancer of the colon and rectum (colorectal cancer) is the most common digestive cancer, and is the second most common cause of cancer death overall in both men and women.

When detected and treated early, digestive cancers are often highly curable. The problem is that these cancers may produce symptoms so vague that the disease often goes undiagnosed until it reaches an advanced stage. In addition, many people don't take advantage of screening tests available to help detect colorectal cancer.

How cancer develops

Simply put, cancer is a clump of abnormal cells. As the cells grow, they form into nodules (tumors) that can press on nerves, block arteries, bleed, obstruct your intestines or interfere with the work of vital organs. Some cancers are slow growing and take years to become life-threatening. Others are fast growing.

No one knows for certain how a normal cell becomes cancerous. A complex mix of factors, including lifestyle, environment and heredity may be responsible. Researchers theorize that most people have dormant genes that can produce cancerous cells. These genes stay dormant until they're activated by an outside agent — such as an infection, sunlight, tobacco or pollutants in food, air or water.

You can get cancer just about anywhere in your digestive tract, but most gastrointestinal cancers occur in the colon and the rectum, where food residue moves more slowly and toxins linger. There are many types of cancer. Those most likely to occur in digestive organs are listed here.

Carcinomas. These are cancers that begin in tissues that line or comprise your internal organs. Most cancers of the digestive system fall into this category.

Lymphomas. These are cancers that develop in your immune system, specifically in your lymph nodes. You have clusters of lymph nodes in your neck, chest, underarms, abdomen and groin. Lymphatic tissue also exists in your intestines and within or near other internal organs.

Sarcomas. These are cancers that start in connective tissues, such as muscle or bone. Smooth muscle exists throughout the digestive tract.

Cancer of the esophagus

Cancer can develop in any part of your esophagus. Researchers aren't certain of its cause, but your risk increases if you smoke or drink excessive amounts of alcohol. Barrett's esophagus, a complication of gastroesophageal reflux disease (GERD), is another known risk factor. (See "Barrett's esophagus" on page 70.) A diet low in fruits and vegetables also appears to increase your risk.

> **Key signs and symptoms**
> - Difficulty swallowing
> - Blood in vomit or stool
> - Weight loss
> - Chest pain

Men are nearly twice as likely to have esophageal cancer as are women. Blacks are three times more likely to have it than are whites.

Estimated new cancer cases and deaths — 2003*

Cancer cases by site and sex

Men	Women
Prostate 220,900	Breast 211,300
Lung & bronchus 91,800	Lung & bronchus 80,100
Colon & rectum 72,800	Colon & rectum 74,700
Urinary bladder 42,200	Uterine corpus 40,100
Non-Hodgkin's lymphoma 28,300	Ovary 25,400
Skin (melanoma) 29,900	Non-Hodgkin's lymphoma 25,100
Oral cavity 18,200	Skin (melanoma) 24,300
Kidney 19,500	Urinary bladder 15,200
Leukemia 17,900	Pancreas 15,800
Pancreas 14,900	Thyroid 16,300
All cancers 675,300	All cancers 658,800

Cancer deaths by site and sex

Men	Women
Lung & bronchus 88,400	Lung & bronchus 68,800
Prostate 28,900	Breast 39,800
Colon & rectum 28,300	Colon & rectum 28,800
Pancreas 14,700	Pancreas 15,300
Non-Hodgkin's lymphoma 12,200	Ovary 14,300
Leukemia 12,100	Non-Hodgkin's lymphoma 11,200
Esophagus 9,900	Leukemia 9,800
Liver 9,200	Uterine corpus 6,800
Urinary bladder 8,600	Brain 5,800
Stomach 7,000	Stomach 5,100
All cancers 285,900	All cancers 270,600

*Excluding basal and squamous cell skin cancers and *in situ* carcinomas, except urinary bladder cancer.

Source: American Cancer Society

Unfortunately, very small tumors in your esophagus usually don't produce any symptoms. Often, the first clue that you have an esophageal tumor is increasing difficulty in swallowing. By this time, however, the cancer may have grown to fill about half the opening of your esophagus. As the cancer becomes advanced, you may experience weight loss, chest pain and blood in your vomit or stool.

There are two common types of esophageal cancer.

Squamous cell carcinoma. This type of cancer forms in flat, scaly (squamous) cells that line the entire length of your esophagus.

Adenocarcinoma. This is cancer in glandular tissue that can develop in your lower esophagus (Barrett's esophagus).

Diagnosis

There are no tests to screen for cancer of the esophagus. If you're experiencing symptoms, you may have a barium X-ray. Just before an X-ray series, you swallow a liquid containing barium, a chalky substance that outlines your esophagus in white. This helps tumors and other abnormalities show up better on the X-ray film.

Endoscopy, a more sensitive test, may be used instead of a barium X-ray, or it may follow a barium X-ray. Your doctor inserts a thin, flexible tube with an attached tiny camera (endoscope) down your throat to look for cancer growth or suspicious tissue.

If you have cancer, blood tests and computerized tomography (CT) or endoscopic ultrasound can help determine how far the cancer has spread. With the latter test, an endoscope containing a small ultrasound probe is placed in your esophagus. The probe releases sound waves that echo off the esophageal walls, creating a computerized picture showing the extent of the cancer on a video monitor.

Treatment

The most common treatment for esophageal cancer is to remove the cancerous section of the esophagus and reconnect the remaining healthy sections. If a large portion of your esophagus is removed, your surgeon may form a new passageway from your throat to your stomach using tissue from a portion of your intestines. Surgery may cure the cancer. Most often, though, it only reduces symptoms and may prolong survival. Eventually, the cancer recurs in most people.

Chemotherapy and radiation are sometimes used, alone or in combination, to ease symptoms, shrink the tumor or kill cancerous cells that have spread from the tumor.

Another treatment method, called photodynamic therapy, uses medications that make the cancer cells sensitive to laser light so that a laser can destroy them. Once esophageal cancer is diagnosed, prognosis often depends on how much the cancer has spread.

Stomach cancer

In the the 1930s, stomach cancer was the leading cause of cancer death among males in the United States. Since then, the incidence of stomach cancer has decreased dramatically. Researchers believe improved methods of food preservation may be the main reason for the decline. Today, most perishable foods are frozen or refrigerated. Years ago, salting and smoking were the common methods for preserving foods — processes that may have lead to formation of cancer-causing substances (carcinogens) in food.

Key signs and symptoms

- Upper abdominal pain
- Nausea and vomiting
- Loss of appetite
- Feeling full after eating only a moderate amount
- Blood in vomit or stool

Improved socioeconomic status and sanitation practices also may be responsible for the decline by reducing the incidence of *Helicobacter pylori (H. pylori)* infection. *H. pylori* is a bacterium associated with peptic ulcers and stomach cancer.

Other factors that may increase risk for stomach cancer include:
- Smoking
- Excessive alcohol use
- Family history of stomach cancer
- Small growths in the stomach lining (adenomatous polyps)
- Previous surgery to remove a portion of your stomach (partial gastrectomy)

- Vitamin B-12 deficiency (pernicious anemia) and associated wasting (atrophy) of the stomach lining

Ninety percent to 95 percent of all stomach cancers form in glandular tissues that line the stomach (adenocarcinomas). Compared with other kinds of cancer, stomach cancer is now uncommon in the United States. However, in developing countries where smoking and salting are still used for food preservation and where *H. pylori* is prevalent, stomach cancer is a leading cause of cancer deaths.

Diagnosis and treatment

A barium X-ray and endoscopy are the most common tests for diagnosing stomach cancer. Endoscopic ultrasound can determine how far the cancer has spread into the stomach wall and adjacent tissues.

There are three main treatments for stomach cancer — surgery, chemotherapy and radiation. The kind of treatment you may receive depends on many factors, including the location and stage of the cancer and your overall health.

Surgery is the only way to cure some stomach cancers. If the cancer is limited to the stomach and nearby lymph nodes, a surgeon may remove the lymph nodes and all or a part of your stomach. If the cancer is advanced, removing a portion of your stomach may relieve signs and symptoms such as vomiting or bleeding.

Chemotherapy and radiation can shrink tumors, which may relieve symptoms and extend your survival. Some studies suggest they may also delay or prevent cancer recurrence after surgery.

When diagnosed and treated early, stomach cancer often can be cured. The prognosis for more advanced cancer depends on the extent of spread of the tumor.

Cancer of the small intestine

This type of cancer is rare. Only about 2 percent of all digestive cancers occur in the small intestine, with 5,300 cases reported yearly in this country. Of these, adenocarcinomas and lymphomas are most common.

The cause of cancer of the small intestine is unknown, but you're at greater risk of having this kind of cancer if you have Crohn's disease or a history of inflammation in the small intestine. The cancer is most often diagnosed in people between the ages of 50 and 60.

Key signs and symptoms
- Cramps
- Bloating
- Nausea and vomiting
- Blood in stool
- Weight loss

Diagnosis and treatment

Cancer of the small intestine typically produces no symptoms in its early stages. The cancer is most often detected in its advanced stages after a barium X-ray series or a CT scan of the small intestine. Depending on the location of the tumor, doctors may be able to see and remove (biopsy) a tissue sample using an endoscope.

The standard treatment is to surgically remove the cancerous tissue. If surgery isn't possible or it fails to stop the cancer from spreading, your doctor may recommend chemotherapy, radiation or both to slow tumor growth and relieve your symptoms. The prognosis for this type of cancer depends on the extent of spread of the tumor.

Gallbladder and bile duct cancers

Also rare, gallbladder cancer occurs in about one in 50,000 Americans, usually women in their 60s and 70s with a history of gallstones. Your risk of gallbladder cancer is four to five times greater if you have gallstones. For uncertain reasons, your risk also seems to be higher the larger your gallstones.

Key signs and symptoms
- Yellowing of skin and eyes (jaundice)
- Abdominal pain
- Nausea
- Fatigue
- Weight loss

About 80 percent of gallbladder cancers are adenocarcinomas. Because early gallbladder cancer causes few symptoms, it's rarely diagnosed in time to cure it. When symptoms do develop, they're generally a result of the cancer invading and obstructing nearby structures, such as the bile ducts, resulting in jaundice.

Cancer of the bile ducts (cholangiocarcinoma) may involve the bile channels within the liver or occur in ducts outside the liver. Primary sclerosing cholangitis, an inflammatory condition affecting the bile ducts often associated with ulcerative colitis, is a known risk factor.

Diagnosis and treatment

Early cancers often are found incidentally during gallbladder surgery to remove gallstones. Ultrasound images can identify gallbladder cancer only about half of the time, often when the disease is in its late stage. Other imaging techniques, such as a computerized tomography (CT) scan, provide little help in finding early cancers, though these tests can help determine how advanced the cancer is.

Removing the gallbladder may cure early cancer. Once the cancer has spread, treatment may focus on relieving your pain and improving your quality of life with medication or radiation.

Cancer of the bile ducts is generally treated with surgery to remove the cancer. Treatment may also include radiation or chemotherapy. If surgery isn't possible, your doctor may place a tiny tube (stent) in the duct to keep it open and relieve jaundice.

The prognosis for gallbladder cancer and cancer of the bile ducts depends on the extent of spread of the tumor.

Liver cancer

Most cancer found in the liver doesn't start there, but spreads there from other locations (secondary or metastatic cancer). Primary cancer that actually starts in the liver is less common.

There are several types of primary liver cancer, but between 70 percent and 85 percent are hepatocellular

Key signs and symptoms
- Abdominal pain
- Weight loss
- Abdominal swelling
- Yellowing of skin and eyes (jaundice)

carcinoma (hepatoma). These are cancers that develop from hepato-cytes, the most common cells in your liver. Researchers theorize that something damages the deoxyribonucleic acid (DNA) of liver cells, causing them to become cancerous.

Liver cancer is two to three times as common in men as in women, and it typically occurs after age 50. These factors may increase your risk:

- Cirrhosis
- Chronic hepatitis B or C infection
- Long-term exposure to aflatoxin, a toxic factor produced by the mold aspergillus
- Exposure to the chemical vinyl chloride used in some plastics
- Long-term use of male hormones that increase muscle mass and strength (anabolic steroids)

Diagnosis

An estimated 17,300 cases of liver cancer were diagnosed during 2003 in the United States. As with most other digestive cancers, liver cancer ordinarily produces few signs and symptoms in its early stages. By the time signs and symptoms emerge, the cancer is often beyond a cure, though not beyond treatment.

Imaging tests of the liver — ultrasound, CT or magnetic reso-nance imaging (MRI) — are generally the first step. If one of these tests suggests cancer, a biopsy of tissue may follow.

Treatment

Surgery is the most effective treatment for liver cancer. If the cancer is small enough, your doctor may be able to remove the tumor and cure the cancer. For a limited group of people who meet specific health criteria, a liver transplant also may be an option. Other treatments for liver cancer often aren't curative, but they may relieve symptoms and extend survival. These include:

- Blocking the blood supply to the tumor by surgically tying the artery that feeds the cancer, or injecting materials that plug up the artery (embolization)
- Blocking the blood supply to the tumor and instilling a chemotherapeutic drug in the sealed-off artery (chemoem-bolization)

- Injecting concentrated alcohol into the tumor to destroy cancer cells (ethanol ablation)
- Destroying the tumor by freezing it (cryosurgery)
- Destroying cancer cells with energy from high-frequency radio waves (radiofrequency ablation)

Traditional chemotherapy and radiation may temporarily shrink liver tumors, but these therapies generally don't help people live much longer. The prognosis for liver cancer depends on the extent of spread of the tumor.

Cancer of the pancreas

Though cancer of the pancreas accounts for only about 2 percent of all new cancer cases in the United States, it's the fourth-leading cause of cancer death. The reason it's so deadly is that it's usually diagnosed too late. The cancer typically produces no signs or symptoms until it's advanced and incurable.

Key signs and symptoms

- Abdominal and/or back pain
- Weight loss
- Yellowing of skin and eyes (jaundice)

In addition, your pancreas is located deep in your abdomen behind other organs, making it impossible for your doctor to detect a lump by feeling (palpating) the area. About 95 percent of pancreas cancers are adenocarcinomas that develop in the lining of pancreatic ducts and may grow undetected for a long time.

Researchers are making progress in understanding how DNA changes may lead to cancer of the pancreas. But much about how or why this cancer develops is still unclear. Several factors may increase your risk.

Smoking. Tobacco use has been determined to be the most important risk factor for pancreatic cancer.

Diet. The second most important risk factor for pancreatic cancer is a diet high in fat and protein.

Family history. Cancer of the pancreas seems to run in families.

Age. Most people are in their 60s and 70s when the disease is diagnosed.

Race. Blacks are more likely to get pancreatic cancer than are other races.

Alcohol. Some studies suggest that excessive alcohol use may increase your risk. Other studies don't confirm this. More research is needed.

Chronic pancreatitis. Most people with long-term inflammation of the pancreas (pancreatitis) don't get cancer of the pancreas, but some do. Why is uncertain.

Diagnosis and treatment

The most common diagnostic tests for detecting pancreatic cancer are ultrasound, CT and MRI. If test results suggest cancer, the next step may be an ultrasound-guided needle biopsy to remove tissue samples. Tissue samples may also be obtained using a long, flexible tube with attached cutting tools (endoscope). The endoscope is inserted into your mouth and threaded through your esophagus and stomach to your upper small intestine (duodenum), where the pancreas excretes its chemicals.

If the cancer is confined to your pancreas, surgically removing all or part of your pancreas can occasionally lead to a cure. The Whipple procedure is the most common surgical procedure. This operation removes part of your pancreas, part of your stomach and the first portion of your small intestine, along with all of your gall-bladder and part of your common bile duct. It's a difficult operation. In large hospitals where surgeons are experienced in the procedure, fewer than 5 percent of the people die of surgical complications. In smaller hospitals, the mortality rate is higher. Radiation and chemotherapy may help extend survival, but they don't cure cancer of the pancreas. The prognosis for more advanced cancer depends on the extent of spread of the tumor.

Cancer of the colon and rectum

Of all digestive cancers, cancer of the colon and rectum (colorectal cancer) is the most common. In 2003, about 147,500 cases of colorectal cancer were diagnosed in the United States. Unlike most other digestive cancers, the long-term survival rate is good, provided the disease is caught early. The five-year survival rate for people with early-stage colorectal cancer is about 90 percent.

Key signs and symptoms

- Blood in stool
- Change in bowel habits
- Abdominal pain
- Weight loss

Screening tests can help detect colorectal cancer in its early stages. However, many people don't take advantage of the tests. That's partly why colorectal cancer caused an estimated 57,000 deaths in the United States in 2003, trailing only lung cancer as a leading cause of cancer death. Once colorectal cancer spreads to adjacent organs or lymph nodes, the five-year survival rate declines.

Are you at risk?

As with many other digestive cancers, genetics and lifestyle appear to play important roles in the development of colorectal cancer.

Family history. You have a greater than average risk of getting colorectal cancer if others in your family have it. All forms of colorectal cancer have a genetic basis.

One type of inherited cancer is called hereditary nonpolyposis colorectal cancer (HNPCC) syndrome. If you have this syndrome, you have a 50 percent chance of passing the gene to each of your children. You also have between a 70 percent and 85 percent chance of having colon cancer, and at a younger age. The average age of cancer diagnosis among people with HNPCC is mid-40s, compared with 65 years for a person with noninherited colorectal cancer.

Another inherited condition is familial adenomatous polyposis (FAP), which produces hundreds, even thousands, of small precancerous growths (polyps) in your colon and rectum. The polyps typically first appear in your teenage years. If FAP isn't diagnosed and the colon removed, cancer almost always develops in one or more of these polyps, generally by the age of 40.

Colorectal polyps. Nearly all colorectal cancer begin with changes in the intestinal lining (adenomas). These changes appear as noncancerous (benign) polyps. Not all polyps become cancerous, but almost all colon cancers start as polyps (see "Colorectal polyps — Early warning signs" on page 183).

Previous colorectal cancer. New cancers or polyps may develop in other locations in your colon or rectum.

Race. Black men and women are at increased risk of colorectal cancer. For example, in 2000 the incidence of colorectal cancer among blacks was 62.7 cases per 100,000. For whites, the incidence was 52.5 cases per 100,000.

Age. Nine out of 10 people who have colorectal cancer are older than age 50.

History of inflammatory bowel disease. A long-term history of ulcerative colitis or Crohn's disease of the colon increases your risk of colorectal cancer, and of developing it at a younger age.

Smoking. Research shows higher rates of colon cancer among people who smoke tobacco. The longer you smoke and the more tobacco you use, the greater your risk.

Diet. People who eat a high-fat diet, especially one that contains a lot of red meat, such as beef, pork and lamb, have a higher risk. A diet high in fiber, on the other hand, has long been considered a way to lower your risk of colorectal cancer. The role of fiber, however, is controversial. Recent studies suggest that fiber doesn't protect against colorectal cancer.

Exercise. People who are inactive tend to be at increased risk of colorectal cancer. This may be related to obesity because people who are inactive also tend to be overweight.

Symptoms

Symptoms can vary depending on the location and extent of the cancer. A cancer located in the lower colon or rectum can block the passage of stool, causing cramps and making it difficult for you to have a bowel movement. You may frequently feel the urge to have a bowel movement, and even after having it you may still feel the urge. Blood in your stool or in the toilet bowl is another warning sign.

Cancer higher up in your colon can cause anemia and fatigue, due to blood loss that you may not be able to see. The blood is usually mixed in with the stool and dark in color. Other symptoms include persistent diarrhea or constipation, decreased appetite, unexplained weight loss, and abdominal pain.

Screening and diagnosis

A panel of the U.S. Preventive Services Task Force has strongly recommended that most people begin colorectal cancer screening at age 50. If you have a family history of colorectal cancer or polyps, or if you have inflammatory bowel disease, you may want to start screening earlier.

Many tests are available to monitor the health of your colon and rectum and identify cancer. They include:
- Colonoscopy
- Sigmoidoscopy
- Colon X-ray (barium X-ray)
- Digital rectal exam
- Fecal occult blood test

Colonoscopy is considered the gold standard for colon cancer detection. During this procedure, a thin, flexible tube with an attached camera is inserted into your rectum and threaded through the colon. The procedure allows your doctor to look for cancer or precancerous polyps. Detection and removal of polyps reduce your chance of having colon cancer by more than 90 percent. An alternative to colonoscopy is sigmoidoscopy combined with a colon X-ray.

Treatment

Surgery and chemotherapy are the two main treatments for colon cancer. Rectal cancer has the same treatment options plus radiation therapy. Depending on the type of cancer you have (colon or rectal), your general health, and the size, location and extent of the tumor, you may have just one or all three forms of therapy.

Surgery often is the treatment of choice because of the various procedures available and their success rates. If the cancer is small, your surgeon may be able to remove it during colonoscopy (polypectomy). Otherwise, your surgeon will make an incision in your abdomen and remove the cancerous portion of the colon, along with some healthy colon on each side. The surgeon may also remove

Colorectal polyps — Early warning signs

The lining inside your colon and rectum is usually smooth. But some people have polyps, mushroom-like growths that sprout up from the lining and intrude into the channel through which food waste passes. Most people with polyps will have one or a few at any given time, but some people may have hundreds or thousands.

Your risk of having polyps increases with age. As many as four out of 10 people older than age 60 have polyps. Most polyps don't become cancerous, but some do. The smaller the polyp, the less likely it is to be cancerous. The precancerous stage is your window of opportunity to detect and remove the growths. Your doctor can remove polyps during colonoscopy. A thin wire is passed through a hollow section of the scope to snare the polyp.

You should have a colonoscopy examination, or a sigmoidoscopy examination combined with a colon X-ray, beginning at age 50. Repeat the tests every five years. If you have a higher than average risk of colorectal cancer, your doctor may recommend that screening begin at an earlier age, and that it be done more often.

In an attempt to identify at an even earlier stage people who may be at risk of polyps and subsequent cancer, Mayo Clinic doctors are experimenting with a magnifying lens that's attached to a colonoscope. With the lens — which magnifies up to 100 times normal size — doctors look for cellular pattern changes called aberrant crypt foci (ACF) in the tissue that lines the colon. Researchers are counting the number of ACF they find in study participants to see if a certain number equates to a higher risk of polyps.

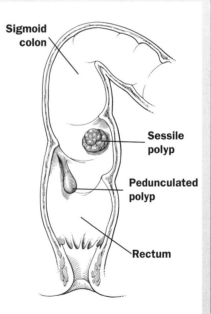

Polyps are small, noncancerous growths of various shapes that may appear in your colon and rectum. Polyps that grow on fleshy stalks are called pedunculated. Those that are flat and have a broad base are sessile polyps.

adjacent tissue containing lymph nodes in an effort to remove microscopic cancer cells that may have migrated from the original tumor.

Another option is laparoscopic surgery. Surgeons remove a portion of your colon through three or four small incisions, instead of one large one. Among surgeons experienced in this technique, laparoscopic surgery has had good results with a shorter hospital stay and, perhaps, less risk of postoperative complications.

Surgery may be followed by radiation or chemotherapy to kill cancerous cells still present after surgery. For advanced cancer that can't be treated surgically, radiation and chemotherapy can help shrink tumors, relieving symptoms and extending survival.

The success of treatment depends on how advanced the cancer is. If the disease is caught early, you have an excellent chance of a cure. Once the cancer spreads to nearby organs and lymph nodes, survival rates decline. Your doctor is best qualified to discuss this with you.

Additional resources

Contact these organizations for more information about digestive conditions. Some groups offer free printed material or videotapes. Others have material or videos you can purchase.

American Cancer Society

1599 Clifton Road, N.E.
Atlanta, GA 30329
(800) ACS-2345, or (800) 227-2345
www.cancer.org

American College of Gastroenterology

P.O. Box 3099
Arlington, VA 22302
(703) 820-7400
www.acg.gi.org

American Dietetic Association

120 S. Riverside Plaza, Suite 2000
Chicago, IL 60606
(800) 877-1600

www.eatright.org

American Gastroenterological Association

4930 Del Ray Ave.
Bethesda, MD 20814
(301) 654-2055
www.gastro.org

American Hemochromatosis Society

4044 W. Lake Mary Blvd.
Unit 104, PMB 416
Lake Mary, FL 32746
(888) 655-4766 or (407) 829-4488
www.americanhs.org

American Institute for Cancer Research

1759 R St. N.W.
Washington, DC 20009
(800) 843-8114 or (202) 328-7744
www.aicr.org

American Liver Foundation

75 Maiden Lane, Suite 603
New York, NY 10038
(800) 465-4837 or (212) 668-1000
www.liverfoundation.org

American Society of Colon and Rectal Surgeons

85 W. Algonquin Road, Suite 550
Arlington Heights, IL 60005
(847) 290-9184
www.fascrs.org

Canadian Celiac Association

5170 Dixie Rd., Suite 204
Mississauga, ON L4W 1E3
Canada
(904) 507-6208 or (800) 363-7296 (Canada only)
www.celiac.ca

Celiac Disease Foundation

13251 Ventura Blvd., #1
Studio City, CA 91604
(818) 990-2354
www.celiac.org

Celiac Sprue Association CSA/USA Inc.

P.O. Box 31700
Omaha, NE 68131
(402) 558-0600
www.csaceliacs.org

Centers for Disease Control and Prevention

1600 Clifton Road
Atlanta, GA 30333
(800) 311-3435
www.cdc.gov

Crohn's and Colitis Foundation of America

386 Park Ave. S.
17th Floor
New York, NY 10016
(800) 932-2423
www.ccfa.org

Gluten Intolerance Group of North America

15110 10th Ave., S.W.
Suite A
Seattle, WA 98166
(206) 246-6652
www.gluten.net

The Hemochromatosis Foundation

P.O. Box 8569
Albany, NY 12208
(518) 489-0972
www.hemochromatosis.org

Hepatitis Foundation International

504 Blick Drive
Silver Spring, MD 20904
(800) 891-0707 or (301) 622-4200
www.hepfi.org

Iron Disorders Institute

P.O. Box 2031
Greenville, SC 29602
(864) 292-1175
www.irondisorders.org

Iron Overload Diseases Association

433 Westwind Drive
North Palm Beach, FL 33408
(561) 840-8512
www.ironoverload.org

International Foundation for Functional Gastrointestinal Disorders

P.O. Box 170864
Milwaukee, WI 53217
(888) 964-2001 or (414) 964-1799
www.iffgd.org

Mayo Clinic Health Information

Mayo Clinic Health Information
200 1st St. S.W.
Rochester, MN 55905
www.MayoClinic.com

National Cancer Institute

Public Inquiries Office
6116 Executive Blvd., MSC8322
Suite 3036A
Bethesda, MD 20892
(800) 4-CANCER, or (800) 426-6237
www.cancer.gov/cancerinfo

National Digestive Disease Information Clearinghouse

2 Information Way
Bethesda, MD 20892
(301) 654-3810 or (800) 891-5389
www.digestive.niddk.nih.gov

National Institute of Diabetes & Digestive & Kidney Diseases

Office of Communications and Public Liaison
NIDDK, NIH
31 Center Dr., MSC 2560
Building 31, Room 9A04
Bethesda, MD 20892
(301) 496-3583
www.niddk.nih.gov

Tri-County Celiac Support Group

TCCSG Shopping Guide
47829 Vistas Circle North
Canton, MI 48188
www.tccsg.com

United Ostomy Association

19772 MacArthur Blvd., Suite 200
Irvine, CA 92612
(800) 826-0826
www.uoa.org

Index